Springer Series on
ADULTHOOD and AGING

Series Editor: Bernard D. Starr, Ph.D.

Advisory Board: Paul D. Baltes, Ph.D., Jack Botwinick, Ph.D.,
Carl Eisdorfer, M.D., Ph.D., Donald E. Gelfand, Ph.D.,
Robert Kastenbaum, Ph.D., Neil G. McCluskey, Ph.D.,
K. Warner Schaie, Ph.D., Nathan W. Shock, Ph.D., and Asher Woldow, M.D.

Virginia C. Little, Ph.D., ACSW, is a professor at the University of Connecticut School of Social Work where she has been a faculty member since 1967. Prior to this she had extensive practice experience in child welfare and mental health, as well as work with the aging. Her doctoral studies at Yale in international relations, and several periods of residence abroad, kindled her interest in comparing service delivery systems in other countries with those in the United States. She has traveled extensively during the past eight years in pursuit of data both in Asia and Europe and has published numerous articles and papers reporting her work.

Dr. Little is a member of the Academy of Certified Social Workers and a Fellow of the Gerontological Society of America. She holds memberships in numerous international organizations and is the only American associate of AGE CONCERN—England and St. James Settlement, Hong Kong.

OPEN CARE FOR THE AGING

Comparative International Approaches

Virginia C. Little

Springer Publishing Company
New York

Springer Publishing Company, Inc.
200 Park Avenue South
New York, New York   10003

82 83 84 85 86 / 10 9 8 7 6 5 4 3 2 1

Library of Congress Cataloging in Publication Data

Little, Virginia C.
  Open care for the aging.

  (Springer series on adulthood and aging; 11)
  Bibliography: p.
  Includes index.
  1. Aged—Services for.   I. Title.   II. Series.
[DNLM: 1. Delivery of health care.   2. Geriatrics.
3. Cross-cultural comparison.   4. Health services
for the aged.   W1 SP685N v. 11 / WT 30 L778o]
HV1451.L57   362.6'3   81-16657
ISBN 0-8261-3750-4   AACR2
ISBN 0-8261-3751-2 (pbk.)

Printed in the United States of America

Contents

Preface

This book has been long in the making. It was conceived in Vienna in 1948 and 1949 when, as a Quaker relief worker, I first undertook the job of service provider. It grew during years of child welfare and mental health work in rural Vermont. As I expanded my horizons to include old people, I encountered the same kinds of service gaps and knee-jerk responses: institutionalize first; provide services later. My hypothesis that this was a problem largely of rural, war-devastated, or underdeveloped areas was shaken when I worked for three years in a major metropolitan area which prided itself on its human services. Where were the services?

When I entered full-time teaching in September 1967, I hoped to bring together my expertise in international relationships with my social work knowledge and skills and concern over delivery systems. In the first seven years I tried numerous avenues and found international conferences to be the most productive of new ideas and new contacts. Hence, beginning in the summer of 1972, I launched myself on a period of travel, field work, and attendance at international meetings on social welfare and gerontology all around the world. For example, the summer of 1972 was devoted to field work and conference attendance in the Soviet Union and the Hague, interspersed with residence in Britain and in West Germany. This was followed in the succeeding summer by travel in Spain and Portugal, which itself preceded a round-the-world sabbatical trip in the academic year 1973–1974, covering some 26 countries.

The pace did not slacken thereafter, but included Far Eastern trips in 1975–1976, a Pacific summer in 1976, European studies in 1977, Far Eastern travels in the summer of 1978, and a semester as visiting professor in Hong Kong in 1978–1979. This made it possible to check preliminary observations and to gather additional data. The two most recent Far

Eastern trips, in 1978 and 1979, have also permitted visits to the People's Republic of China.

Studying aging around the world is not possible without the help and support of many people. I could not possibly list all who have guided, conducted, entertained and supported me. I'm sure to have forgotten some; others are mentioned in my references.

For a combination of financial help and moral support, thanks are due to many. First, to the Gerontological Society of America, beginning with a scholarship to attend a Summer Institute in Gerontology in Asheville, North Carolina in summer 1971; to a Summer Research Fellowship for studying home care in Connecticut in summer 1975; and finally to selection as one of ten United States scholars to receive a travel grant to Japan for a comparative study with Japanese scholars.

Others have helped with work in the Far East. For funding the project in Western Samoa, I owe particular thanks to the Center for Field Research and to Betsy Caney, Research Director. For arranging a consortium of Hong Kong universities and the Department of Social Welfare and Hong Kong Council of Social Service to sponsor my visiting professorship, special thanks to Professor Peter Hodge of the University of Hong Kong. The University of Connecticut Research Foundation has helped with a small grant to finance interviews for the cross-national project with Japan, and with partial travel grants to present papers at national and international meetings, as well as clerical assistance. Also, the University of Hawaii has helped with conference and consultant invitations, and the Asia Foundation underwrote my 1978–1979 travel to Hong Kong.

Finally, special thanks to students, both in the United States and abroad, whose questions and comments have sparked many leads. I am particularly grateful to the three student interviewers in Connecticut: Jean Manix, David Carroll and Kenneth Richard for labor above and beyond the call of duty.

I have tried to express in the dedication my debts to many people. The responsibility for any errors of fact and judgment is, of course, my own.

Part I

Conceptual
Framework

1

Introduction

A World Assembly on Aging is planned for the year 1982. This reflects a growing concern in United Nations circles, as well as in leading countries, about the widening gap between population projections forecasting increases in the numbers and proportion of older people, and the continuum of care available to meet their needs.

A 1973 United Nations report summarized the situation in these terms: the world approaches the year 2000 without a policy on aging, with little planning, and with gaps and fragmentation in both health and social service delivery systems (United Nations, 1973).

Since 1973 there has been some growth in long-term care facilities but the population at risk is growing at a faster rate. No country is fully satisfied with its present services. The hope for the 1982 world meeting, and beyond, is that countries at different stages of development may benefit by sharing their experiences in caring for the frail elderly. Can developing societies find ways to fund and manage formal structures, avoiding some of the dysfunctionalities of bureaucratic systems? Can developed countries revive or shore up family and informal supports? Can both learn from one another in achieving an appropriate service mix?

This is an exploratory study within a stages-of-development framework. The data are drawn from the author's own travel and residence abroad, supplemented by official and private reports, as well as by personal correspondence. It seeks to establish what the present data base is, while calling for an expanded data base, and improved quantitative and qualitative indicators. It examines a variety of approaches, some of which may be considered as models, but is more concerned with fact-finding and analysis than with model building.

3

Who are the aging? How is the population at risk defined? How has the aging of populations come to be viewed as a world social problem? These are some of the questions addressed in this initial chapter.

Who Are the Aging?

The aging are ourselves, our present and future selves. The process of aging is one of change over time. Each of us begins to age at the moment of birth (or conception). We all age at the same rate, 24 hours a day. Hence the conventional measure of aging is *chronological*, from date of birth. In developing countries not yet attuned to calendars and clocks, people's ages are known only approximately. However, every society has some method of age grading, to differentiate younger and older age cohorts.

A second approach (also using numbers) is the *legal* definition of age. Legislative judgments change from time to time, as well as from place to place. Beginning with Bismarck's Germany in 1883, the age of male retirement was arbitrarily established at 65. Lately this definition is being changed in many countries, in favor of more flexible retirement options. However, the right to pass laws officially designating persons of a certain age as old has not been challenged.

Legal/chronological measures have also been found convenient for *administrative* purposes. For example, under the Older Americans Act, age 60 was chosen as the basis for the population formula by which federal funds are distributed to states and Indian tribes. Other laws, such as the Social Security Act, have used different ages. At present some Americans retire from their principal occupations as early as age 45, especially in the armed services or assembly line industries. A few go on to second careers or occupations. Others work part time, including some of the officially retired, although subject to social security penalties if they earn above a stated minimum. The use of age 55 by the American Association of Retired Persons (AARP) suggests that this may be the usual *social* definition, at least among the middle class.

Among professional gerontologists a growing minority now favors a *functional* definition. A person is functionally dependent, regardless of age, when he/she cannot perform unaided the usual activities of daily living, such as walking, climbing stairs, personal care. A functional rating can be used in program planning; the incapacitated elderly can be grouped with other disabled persons of varying ages who are potential claimants for the same services. For older people this might help to reduce pejorative labeling and attitudes of ageism. Those not incapacitated would cease to be stereotyped as sick and dependent, on the road to inevitable death. Individual, group, and cohort differences would be recognized. However, the funding structure of present programs based on legal/chronological definitions, as well as administrative convenience, would be threatened.

Population at Risk

Measures of functional dependence, such as activities of daily living scales, can be combined with chronological/legal/administrative/social definitions to specify more clearly the population at risk and the subgroups at special risk, from which smaller groups are targeted for service provision.

Assuming that resources are limited, the first target group might be the most incapacitated (for example, *bedfast, housebound*). Should there be additional resources, services could next be targeted at those found to be *ambulatory with difficulty*. According to cross-national studies, replicated in six countries by Shanas and associates, this proportion is never more than 25 percent of persons aged 65 and over living in the community (Shanas, 1968, 1971, 1974) (Table 1–1). Viewed cross-sectionally, about three-fourths of the old would not require in-home services at a given time. Viewed longitudinally, persons over 80 are statistically more likely to have

Country	Percent Bedfast (a)	Percent Housebound (b)	Percent Ambulatory With Difficulty (c)	b + c
Denmark	2	8	14	22
Britain	3	11	8	19
United States	2	6	6	12
Israel	2	13	NA	NA
Poland	4	6	16	22
Yugoslavia	3	4	20	24

Source: Shanas, E. Health Status of Older People. Cross-national Implications. *American Journal of Public Health*, 1974, 63, 3, 261-264. Reprinted by permission of the author and publisher.

TABLE 1–1. Proportion of Population Aged 65 and Over, Bedfast, Housebound, and Ambulatory Only with Difficulty, in Six Countries

one or more disabilities. Sir Ferguson Anderson, in a paper presented in Kyoto, Japan in August 1978, estimated that only 12 percent of persons aged 65–69 need help, by comparison with 80 percent of those aged 85.

Based on these facts, a population at special risk has been identified as those aged 80 plus, sometimes termed "frail elderly." Not all are frail, but a higher proportion are likely to be. Within this special population are subgroups experiencing additional deprivations, such as substandard income, inadequate housing, poor physical and/or mental health. Minority elderly, although fewer in number, are often in multiple jeopardy. An additional risk factor, often found in developed countries, is that about one-fifth of the oldest survivors are alone, lacking family supports.

Weighing all these factors, Neugarten (1975) proposed that two generations of old people be distinguished: the *young-old* and the *old-old*. Others have elaborated this concept to include additional classes, such as the *middle-aged old* and the *very-old old*. The ages attached to these categories varies somewhat with different users, depending on which age is chosen for a starting point, and whether a ten- or fifteen-year interval is used. My preference is to define them as follows: *young-old*, aged 55–69; *middle-aged old*, 70–84; *old-old*, 85–99; and *very old-old*, 100 or more.

Aging as a Social Problem

Growing old or very old may or may not be a problem for the individual. The aging of populations, however, is now seen as a social problem, both for developed and developing countries, and has been so designated in a series of United Nations reports (1973, 1975, 1978). Not all countries are equally aware of the dimensions of the problem.

Aging has not always been viewed as problematic. There appears to be a poor fit between industrialization, modernization, and aging; in a modern industrialized country more people live longer and require more care over a longer period of retirement. In Japan, where the process is occurring at a faster rate than in older industrial societies, there is growing concern over what Japanese call the "era of man-made longevity." In nonindustrial societies, by contrast, Cowgill and Holmes (1972) gathered evidence that, when the old are fewer in number and still perform valued functions, their status is higher. In primitive societies that are short of food and other resources, Simmons found (1945) that the old are left to die, as a matter of necessity.

In the United States aging was first labelled as a social problem in 1909, in the report of a Massachusetts commission. It was not always so. In colonial America the old were dominant and wigs were worn to affect an older appearance. According to Fisher (1977), however, the social (and later the psychological) status of the old began to diminish even before the technological revolution ushered in by the Civil War.

Do the aging view themselves as a problem? To the extent that they internalize societal values such as independence and "not being a burden," yes. However, as we observe leaders like Maggie Kuhn of the Gray Panthers in action, it appears that organized groups of older people are taking a hand in redefining the situation.

Demographic Projections

The definition of aging as a world social problem rests its case largely on population projections. All of the people who will be old in the year 2000 are already alive. How many will survive to various ages depends on how closely one can estimate age-specific mortality rates. Neugarten presents two estimates, one based on the assumption that they will remain the same; the second that the rates may improve two percent annually, with less cigarette smoking, improved nutrition, and better health habits (Table 1–2).

United Nations projections make the same point: in every country the numbers and proportions of old people, in particular the old-old, will increase. Even for the developing nations where the percentage increases may look small, as in India or Indonesia, the population base is so large that there will be many more in need of long-term care (United Nations, 1978) (Table 1–3).

		1975[a]		2000(A)[a]		2000(B)[b]	
		M	F	M	F	M	F
Total	55+	18.0	23.2	19.7	27.5	24.8	32.4
	65+	8.9	12.8	10.2	16.3	14.4	20.8
	75+	3.1	5.2	4.0	7.7	6.9	11.2
	55–75	14.9	18.0	15.7	19.8	17.9	21.2

[a] If age-specific death rates continue as of 1968

[b] If age-specific death rates are reduced by 2% per year after 1970 for all persons aged 20+

Source: Neugarten, B. L. The Future and the Young-Old. Gerontologist, 1975, 15, I, Part II, 4-10.
Reprinted by permission.

TABLE 1-2. Numbers of Older Persons in the United States in 1975 and in 2000 (in millions)

TABLE 1-3. The 60-and-Over and 80-and-Over Age Groups, Numbers (in thousands) and as Percentages of all Ages, as well as Percent Change, 1970 and 2000, by Regions of the World

Region	Age	1970 Number	1970 Percentage of All Ages	2000 Number	2000 Percentage of All Ages	Percent Change 1970–2000
Africa	All Ages	351,727	100.0	813,681	100.0	+131.3
	60 and Over	16,704	4.7	42,133	5.2	+152.2
	80 and Over	1,235	.35	2,629	.32	+112.9
Latin America	All Ages	283,020	100.0	619,929	100.0	+119.0
	60 and Over	16,483	5.8	41,529	6.7	+152.0
	80 and Over	1,225	.43	3,865	.62	+215.5
Northern America	All Ages	226,389	100.0	296,199	100.0	+30.8
	60 and Over	31,276	13.8	42,965	14.5	+37.4
	80 and Over	3,573	1.6	7,012	2.4	+96.2
East Asia	All Ages	926,866	100.0	1,307,061	100.0	+47.8
	60 and Over	78,331	8.5	157,772	11.5	+101.4
	80 and Over	3,913	.42	8,479	.65	+116.7
South Asia	All Ages	1,101,199	100.0	2,267,266	100.0	+105.9
	60 and Over	53,997	4.9	137,445	6.1	+154.5
	80 and Over	3,622	.33	8,479	.37	+134.1
Europe	All Ages	459,085	100.0	539,500	100.0	+17.5
	60 and Over	76,449	16.7	99,947	18.5	+30.7
	80 and Over	8,118	1.7	13,181	2.4	+62.4
Oceania	All Ages	19,323	100.0	32,715	100.0	+69.3
	60 and Over	2,081	10.8	3,632	11.1	+74.5
	80 and Over	233	1.2	438	1.3	+88.0
U.S.S.R.	All Ages	242,768	100.0	315,027	100.0	+29.8
	60 and Over	29,018	12.0	56,007	17.8	+93.0
	80 and Over	2,920	1.2	7,085	2.2	+142.6

Source: Population by Sex and Age for Regions and Countries, 1950–2000, as Assessed in 1973: Medium Variant (U.N., ESA/P/WP60, 25 February 1976).

2

The Continuum of Care: Defining a Service System

The chief response to the perceived problem of aging has been symbolic, the concept of a "continuum of care." Ideally, this continuum includes a "range of institutions" and a "spectrum of services." With regard to the former, Reader (1972, 1973) listed a dozen types of institutions for geriatric care:

Category of Care	Example
1. home health care	visiting nurses, as in New England
2. day care	geriatric day hospitals as in Britain
3. infirmary care	adjuncts to nursing homes
4. nursing and boarding homes	extended and intermediate care facilities; community care homes
5. chronic disease hospitals	tuberculosis, heart, atherosclerosis
6. geriatric hospitals	as in the United Kingdom
7. terminal care/hospices	St. Christopher's, London
8. mental hospitals	state and county, United States
9. community care for mentally ill	special villages, as in Holland
10. specialty/rehabilitation hospitals	Burke Rehabilitation Center, New York
11. community mental health centers	United States, post–1963
12. short-stay hospitals (acute)	general hospitals, United States and elsewhere

By contrast to the "range of institutions," the "spectrum of services" is

9

broader in scope, and oriented to community-based programs. Looking at the Older Americans Act of 1965, as amended, one finds that "services" include every known social, environmental, health, mental health, legal, transportation, nutrition, employment, recreational, educational, or related service, plus others which may be added in the future. The stated goal is a "comprehensive and coordinated service system for older Americans."

I prefer to use a systems model which places both institutions and services in a wheel rotating around the population at risk. The wheel rests on a tripartite foundation of income maintenance, housing and health care.

The foundation concept was proposed earlier by Kahn and Kamerman (1975). In their most recent formulation (1977), they have added employment and education as additional systems, making the personal social services the sixth system. When there are gaps or deficits in the foundation, the wheel may grind to a halt, like a car with a flat tire.

Open, Closed, and Unorganized Care

The circular systems model depicts what I see as the three major components of the care system: *open, closed,* and *unorganized* care. My terminology is drawn from current studies by the European Centre for Social Welfare Training and Research; it is useful because of the analogy with the terminology of open and closed systems. It also draws attention to the importance of the unorganized or informal sector which, according to current thinking, provides the bulk of the services which older people actually get.

Open care is care in the community, encompassing all of the programs aimed at supporting living in one's own home, and forestalling premature or unnecessary institutionalization. *Closed* care, by contrast, is care in institutions, behind closed doors, including both medical facilities and boarding homes. In closed care there are typically few interchanges with other systems, and a weak or nonexistent feedback loop. The third term, *unorganized* (or nonorganized) is reserved for informal support systems or, to use current jargon, so-called "natural networks"; these include family, relatives, neighbors, friends, community caretakers and irregular volunteers. Regular or organized volunteers would be considered part of the formal structure of either open or closed care.

The boundaries between the three sectors are shifting and are not always seen in the same way. In Sweden, for example, pensioners who live in service houses (residential hotels) are considered to be living in the community. In Austria, however, a leading expert classes the so-called

Pensionistenheime (apartment hotels) in Vienna as part of closed care (Amann, 1980). Similar questions could be raised about the whole range of intermediate housing, such as sheltered flats, "granny flats," warden-supervised old age homes, or the so-called "hostels" in Hong Kong housing estates. I prefer to use the term "open" for all situations in which people are free to come and go as they choose, following their personal preferences for meals, sleeping, recreation and other activities. The term "closed" is then used for settings in which the daily routines are administratively scheduled and enforced; even an understaffed and poorly managed old age home has this characteristic.

There is also question about using the term "unorganized" care for a society which to date has little or no formal care structure, but does have aspirations for the future. Looking at family care in Greece, the same Austrian expert suggests that it is in transition, beginning to look toward open care, of which family care is the precursor. This is correct in that it suggests that most open care services (and closed care) begin as family substitutes. Again, I prefer to use the term "unorganized" for a pre-open care stage of development. When volunteers are organized, as in the United States, for example, so that one obtains a voluntary friendly visitor under a purchase of service contract with a family agency, then I view this as part of formal open care. Similarly, Red Cross and other volunteers who work in American hospitals under the supervision of a paid director of volunteers are considered by me to be a part of closed care.

Nature and Characteristics of the Service System

Present open and closed care programs have been put in place as vaguely conceived family substitutes, when informal supports are deficient. Just as children lacking parents were once placed in orphan asylums, so old persons without families are put away in institutions. There has been little attention to the specific service requirements of the population at risk. The medical acute-care model is widely considered inappropriate for chronic long-term cases, but nevertheless predominates. In the community most services for the old are pale imitations of services for children, e.g., group meals, foster homes, day care centers; one could add birthday and Christmas parties, and trips to scenic and historic sites, summer camps and schools. Can this tendency be explained by a shared stereotype of old age as a second childhood, or simply by lack of imagination?

The word "service" is itself a loose expression, which covers almost any kind of task or transaction. In terms of economic development the distinction is made between *primary* production, or extraction of products from the land by farming and mining; *secondary*, the processing of raw materials by manufacturing and industry; and *tertiary*, or service occupations, which "cover the waterfront," including health/medical, banking, insurance, public employment, private utilities, as well as waiters, barbers, hairdressers, salespeople, and the like. "Public" services can also mean utilities such as gas, water, electricity; police and fire protection; garbage collection and sanitation; plus others performed by faceless bureaucrats.

The term "social services" is even more vague. Are they services performed by "social workers," as the song suggests? Is there a difference between "social services," human services," and/or "personal social services"? If economics is defined as "what economists talk about with one another," then "social" becomes a residual item, somehow related to society, covering what economists do not (or do not yet) discuss. Perhaps the term is deliberately kept vague so that its meaning may be adjusted as circumstances change.

More important for our purposes, is there a *service system* for the vulnerable elderly? A service system, like any system, may be small, medium-sized, or large; familial, local, regional, national, or international. It may include professional, subprofessional and nonprofessional workers; both instrumental ("hard") and expressive ("soft") services. Some may be delivered directly, face-to-face, or by telephone in a worker-client interaction; others may be indirect, such as consultation or case management.

A system is not a system unless it defines its boundaries, states its goals and objectives and analyzes its resources and environmental constraints; it should have at least rudimentary feedback and communications channels (Churchman, 1968).

From a strict point of view, there is serious question whether there is a *system* of social services in the United States. If so, it is one which, according to Kamerman and Kahn (1976), is characterized by gaps, fragmentation, lack of communication, and often by failure to define goals. Because of its lack of systemic essentials, I prefer to characterize it as a *non-system*, although it may be useful at times to assume the potential existence of a system.

Older Americans usually see it as a non-system. The majority have not received any social service, and associate the term with the depression and welfare, "poor services for poor people."

Gilbert and Specht have suggested (1974) that the delivery of services is variously organized, according to a series of basic policy choices, along four dimensions: allocation, provision, delivery, and finance. Administrative organization, management, auspices, financing are diverse, especially in a pluralistic society like the United States; typically, the form is bureaucratic, the variance being explained largely by the size of the unit, the auspices (public, private, proprietary), and the funding sources. Some agencies can be comprehended only as products of their own idiosyncratic histories and the kinds of personalities chosen for management roles. In addition, the terrain is strewn with the remains or wreckage of past demonstration projects, not all of which expand available services.

In designing programs for aging populations at risk, the key issues to be faced are political or allocative. In addition to "how much," and "how good," we need to ask a series of questions:

1. *who delivers* the service: family, friend, volunteer, paraprofessional, professional; uni-, multi-, or inter-disciplinary team;

2. *where* is the service delivered: in the home, a closed care institution, medical facility, congregate meal site, agency office, neighborhood center, senior center, mobile van, or other place;

3. *when* is the service delivered: 24-hour, 7-day week, office hours only, specified client days or times, by appointment only, *ad hoc*, emergency.

4. *who receives* the service: age limits, income limits (means test or sliding scale), sex, race, residence, disability, other eligibility requirements, knowledge limits.

Included in (4) above are *who finds access to* the system (most elderly never do), plus *who drops out*, or *is rejected*. The ultimate question is, of course *who pays*. In the United States and elsewhere, the flow of services follows the flow of funds, and dries up when the money supply is turned off.

Still, we have failed to pinpoint the essential characteristics of a "service" from the standpoint of the potential older consumer. One thumbnail phrase (said to have originated in Finland) is: "anything that doesn't involve giving out money." An American social work point of view has been that services should not be forced on welfare recipients receiving financial aid, hence the separation of eligibility and services. The counterargument, for viewing money payments as a kind of financial service, is that this may in fact be the only aid most people receive, in societies as different as Hong Kong and the United States.

What Is a "Unit of Service"?

If the word "service" is not clearly defined, what then is a "unit of service"? For reimbursement reasons, this has been approached in the United States as a question of quantifying transactions. A unit may vary from a concrete input, such as one hour of home health time, or one round trip to and from a clinic, to one hour of counselling, or one telephone call. If services are quantified largely in units of time, as these examples would suggest, then the most expensive in budgetary terms are those performed by the most highly trained professionals. The least expensive in terms of hourly rates are those performed by an unpaid family member.

Difficulty in conceptualizing the "service system" in other than symbolic or vague phrases renders the delivery of services problematic and leaves the burden of older care where it has always been, with the unorganized sector.

3

Stages of Development

Failure to conceptualize and define the boundaries of a service system has resulted in a hodgepodge of services and programs. Unorganized, closed and open care coexist everywhere. The mix at any moment reflects a myriad of historical, political, economic, and social factors, all of which impinge on current decisions about resource allocation. An overlay of traditional and emerging values, myths, stereotypes and belief systems enriches the rhetoric and obscures the decisional process. Where is a society at a given time in relation to other societies, and in relation to itself at a previous time? What trends can be discerned in developed and developing countries?

I suggest seeking answers to these questions in a stages-of-development framework. If we view the modern welfare state as the product of industrial society, we may then arrange developing and developed countries along a residual-institutional continuum, as proposed by Wilensky and Lebeaux (1967). Looking at a range of services for the elderly, I originally constructed a model with four major stages: *residual, early institutional, institutional,* and *maximum institutional* (Little, 1974). This earlier model focused on the concomitant development of a number of formal programs to supplement continuing family care and natural networks support (Table 3–1).

Using these criteria, I then arranged 24 countries at various stages along a continuum of development (Table 3–2).

These 24 countries were then dichotomized into two groups: Group 1—Developing and Group 2—Developed, as follows:

Group 1—Developing: Afghanistan, Indonesia, Western Samoa, Burma, Pakistan, Kenya, Iran, India, Philippines, Greece, Singapore, Hong Kong.

RESIDUAL: Characterized by:

    1. Family and mutual aid only; some volunteers;
    2. Some private homes for the aged;
    3. No public funding of facilities for the aged;
    4. Lack of training programs;
    5. Lack of home help or other domiciliary services.

EARLY INSTITUTIONAL: Characterized by:

    1. Organized social services, including volunteer organizations;
    2. Attempt at supervision/regulation of private homes;
    3. Some public funding of institutions for the aged;
    4. Professional training programs with an aging component;
    5. Demonstration home help-domiciliary services.

INDICATIVE INSTITUTIONAL: Characterized by:

    1. Specialized medical facilities, such as geriatric hospitals;
       chronic care and attention homes;
    2. Licensing and regulation of private homes by a public agency;
    3. Public funding extended to special housing, community centers,
       and other facilities;
    4. Substantial development of professional training programs;
    5. Substantial development of a range of domiciliary services,
       including home help, Meals on Wheels, laundry, transportation,
       and the like.

MAXIMUM INSTITUTIONAL: Characterized by:

    1. A range of specialized facilities, including day care centers
       and hospitals, halfway houses;
    2. Participation/leadership in regional/international programs
       for establishing and enforcing standards;
    3. Active organization of the aging, political and otherwise;
    4. Regional centers for research, training and community service
       in gerontology;
    5. A cluster of domiciliary services, coordinated with other
       health and welfare subsystems.

Source: Little, V. C. Social Services for the Elderly: With Special
        Attention to the Asia and West Pacific Region (1974).

TABLE 3–1. Specialized Services for the Elderly: Stage of Development Model

Group 2—Developed: New Zealand, Australia, Austria, Germany, Netherlands, United States, Japan, Israel, Canada, Great Britain, Denmark, Sweden.

Initial review of the 24-country data, confirmed by additional study trips and correspondence, suggested four overall hypotheses (Little, 1975a):

1. In every country, a substantial but unmeasured quantity of service is given by families and relatives, supplemented by neighbors, friends and volunteers.

2. In every country there are some institutions such as private homes for old people who lack family support: (a) with few exceptions, there are different kinds of accommodation for those who can afford to pay.

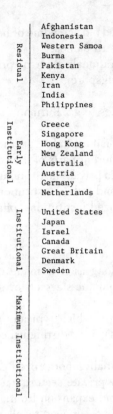

Source: Little, V. C. Field Data.

TABLE 3–2. The Residual-Institutional Continuum of Elderly Services

3. The public provision of institutional care generally precedes that of community care, and its funding tends to be at a higher level, at every stage of economic and social development.

4. Home-delivered services to supplement family care are seriously deficient, and in most countries available only on a minimal basis, justifying the appellation "Cinderella services."

Additional countries since visited have enriched but have not altered the basic concept. Further support for a stages-of-development approach has come from analysis of presently available data on the three components of care.

Closed care usually develops first. I have identified six different levels, the first three characteristic of developing countries and the second of more developed countries (Little, 1979a). The six levels are:

Level 1: privately sponsored old age home or homes, often by church or religious bodies, e.g., Western Samoa;

Level 2: regulation and rationalization of private homes to meet community standards, e.g., Singapore;

Level 3: model homes,

    (a) semi-public auspices, e.g., Burma:

    (b) public,

        (1) one in the national capital, e.g., the Philippines;

        (2) five or six in different parts of the country, e.g. Thailand;

Level 4: public payments to private institutions, e.g., United States;

Level 5: a mix of private and public institutions, e.g., Japan;

Level 6: a range of specialized institutions, offering various levels of care, e.g., Britain.

For convenience these stages may also be viewed as a continuum from less to more public provision, as long as it is made clear that there is no necessary linear progression from one stage or level to the next. Fixation and regression may also occur.

Similarly, within *open care*, which typically develops after closed care, at least four different levels may be distinguished, and a possible fifth:

Level 1: embryonic, essentially unorganized care;

Level 2: emergent, largely private sector;

Level 3: rapid transition and expansion from a public welfare base;

Level 4: extension of public services to all parts of the country, including rural areas.

These four levels parallel the four stages of development previously proposed, and are useful for a closer examination of the service system, or non-system, of a given country.

There is also a possible fifth level, that of coordination and integration of services. Again, because growth is not necessarily linear, the coordination/integration problem may be identified before an adequate base of direct services is developed as, for example, in the United States.

In Part Two, which follows, Western Samoa has been chosen as an example of Level 1, Hong Kong of Level 2, Japan of Level 3, and Sweden of Level 4. Presentation of data on their mix of services will be followed by an examination of the major issues and problems which occur at all levels: the family as a unit of care; the quantity and quality of services provided (level of effort), assessing needs; and coping with the complexities of a mature system.

Part II
The Care Mix in Four Different Societies

4

Western Samoa:
Level 1

It is not easy to find a "pure" example of unorganized care in the modern world. A country like Afghanistan is undeveloped, but also lacks data. Western Samoa has been chosen because some data are available from a multidisciplinary team research project conducted in the summer of 1976, which shed light on an early stage of development: the introduction of the first old-age home, sponsored by a Roman Catholic order, the Little Sisters of the Poor, which opened its doors in April, 1975.

Since my report of the preliminary data from the 1976 project (Little, 1976), interest has flared up in what is now being called "the coming of old age in Samoa" and a comparable study, replicating some of my findings, has been done by Cernak (1979).

Samoa is a good example of how difficult it is to break the barrier of myths and stereotypes, in this case about the islands, as well as about aging. Almost everyone has read Margaret Mead (1928). The adolescents whom Mead studied in the 1920s are now septenarians and in their lifetimes they have experienced major political, economic and social changes which have impacted their traditional culture. Some have died, while others survive to tell the tale.

Additional reasons why Western Samoa makes a good case study of changing eldercare include:

1. It has a largely undeveloped economy, just beginning to enter the modern world of money wages.
2. Unlike American Samoa, a United States dependency, it has been independent since January 1, 1962. It still retains ties with the former trust country, New Zealand, in particular the continuing out-migration of the young and economically active to New Zealand for paid employment.

3. The extended family *(aina)* survives, eroded by migration of the young, but sustained in part by the money remittances they send from abroad.

4. The country has no scheme of public welfare, no public social insurance, and no private charities, other than the old-age home.

Background

Western Samoa, with an area of 1,100 square miles, lies in central Polynesia, and consists of two main islands, Savaii and Upolu, and seven smaller islands. Somewhat analogously to the Hawaiian Islands, Savai'i is the "Big Island," whereas the capital city, Apia, is located on Upolu.

The total population is now about 175,000 people, some 40,000 of whom live in Apia. Nine out of 10 are full Samoans. Less than three percent are age 65 or over; thus, the age structure is young, according to United Nations guidelines. There is a gap in presently aging cohorts, especially males, attributable to the high death rate from the influenza epidemic at the close of the First World War.

The true birth rate is estimated at 35/1,000 and the crude death rate at 7/1,000. The rate of natural increase is therefore a little less than three percent annually. The estimated out-migration (mainly to New Zealand) is between 3,500 and 4,000 persons annually. The life expectancy for females is given as 63.8 years; for males, 60.8 (Western Samoa, Health Statistics, 1977).

Health

Higher life expectancy than that reported for many developing countries reflects favorable climatic and food conditions more than it does resource allocation to the health and medical sector. The present medical care system continues the colonial-type model established during the New Zealand trusteeship, with a base hospital in the capital city of Apia to which patients may be transported, by air if necessary, for more specialized care and attention. This is supplemented by a few district hospitals on the other islands, which usually have minimal budgets and are weakly staffed by trained medical personnel. There is also a network of district nurses with multiple duties, including working with traditional women's committees to improve sanitation and unorganized care in the villages. The Apia general hospital is reported to have a 75 percent bed occupancy rate, whereas other hospitals are under 30 percent and frequently about 20 percent (Western Samoa, Review of the Economy, 1977).

Persons entering a hospital receive medical attention but, especially in district hospitals, are cared for principally by relatives, who provide food, clothing, bedding, laundry service, personal care, and companionship. Going to a hospital is a last resort when all else fails, as is going to a dentist. Most older people extract their own bad teeth, and for other complaints rely on home remedies, such as *ti*-leaves, or tying rags around the hurting part. This may be supplemented by a massage either by a family member or a local specialist, the *fofo*.

The village women's committees are now the custodians of a small amount of drugs and medication supplied by the district nurse and, between her visits, dispensed according to their best judgment. Some people buy aspirin-type products at the local store. Only one or two in the sub-villages studied in the project had access to other aids, such as eyeglasses; an available pair of glasses was shared with relatives and friends. Those having mobility problems (as many do) relied on walking sticks picked up in the environs.

Although there is a psychiatric ward in the Apia hospital, there are no mental institutions. The nonviolent are cared for at home by family members; the violent are incarcerated in jails with criminals.

Housing

In Apia there are still examples of older colonial housing, gracious mansions with wide verandas, some dating back to the German time (pre-1914). When one flies over the islands in a small airplane, one sees from the air many rusting corrugated shacks, also dating back to earlier times. However, the majority of Samoans continue to occupy open *fales,* with thatched roofs and no sides, except for handwoven blinds which can be lowered in case of rain. The dirt floors are covered with mats woven by the women. Dogs, cats, poultry and people wander freely in and out.

Cooking is done outdoors, usually under a roof, and there is a big oven where such larger items as pigs may be roasted for a feast or for Sunday. Personal washing and laundry are done outdoors, often in the sea. There are now enclosed latrines, part of the government's public health campaign, although one still sees old outhouses at the end of piers stretching over the water, another relic of the German era.

An older couple typically lives in a separate *fale*, close to those of relatives, who visit frequently and bring prepared food. The *fales* close to the main road tend to be neat and in good repair; those farther back in the forest are less so. When able, older people tidy up their own huts on the inside, and cut the grass and vines in the immediately surrounding area.

Income Maintenance

People work on the plantations and fish as long as they feel able, then gradually phase themselves out in favor of remaining at home. Food is plentiful and clothing simple, usually consisting of a single piece of cloth *(lava-lava)*; more elaborate costumes to wear to church on Sunday are carefully preserved in chests in mothballs. Shoes are seldom used, except for simple plastic thongs, generally imported from Japan.

Those who need help turn first to family members, even to relatives in other villages. Church members, led by the pastor and church women's committees, are active in home visiting and offering support. However, my own observation in the 1976 project, which included interviews with community leaders as well as with old people, was that the informal support system, although available, provided little in the way of actual financial, material, or other hard services, and functioned more as a method of social control. Individuals interviewed were reluctant to ask for help, which appeared to be stigmatized in a way analogous to applying for welfare elsewhere (Little, 1976).

In the three sub-villages we studied, there was increasingly heavy reliance on remittances from abroad, largely from New Zealand. There was a noticeable decline of involvement in plantation farming and fishing; instead, people preferred to stop in the local store and buy a tin of bully beef or a can of sardines. Although there is a publicized government-sponsored National Provident Fund, in which individuals are invited to deposit their savings, there were only two families which reported having made deposits.

The Care System

There is no formal system of social welfare or social services. The main target of government's five-year development plan is economic growth. Small symbolic gestures are made in favor of nutrition and health education, mainly by the district nurses. The overall assumption has been that formal social services are not needed, since the extended family will take care of children, the aged, and other vulnerable groups who need assistance. This assumption is questioned not only by the findings of our project, but also by the success of the first old age home, Mapuifagelele.

Closed Care

When the home first opened its doors in 1975, this was the culmination of a lengthy campaign led by the highly respected local Roman Catholic cardinal. Nursing sisters of the order known as the Little Sisters of the Poor were assigned to Apia, and cared for many old people in the community for three years before the building was ready for occupancy.

The building itself was funded in part by the international order and in part by local donations, at an estimated cost of $1.5 million (Australian). No fees are charged, as this order relies on donations to continue its work. The age of eligibility for admission is 60; priority is given to those who need medical care, regardless of religion or place of residence.

The most recent census is given as 83 residents, 38 male and 45 female. The average age is 76; the oldest resident is 98. As in any home for old people, the census changes as some patients die and others are admitted.

I studied a total of 92 cases, encompassing all admissions from the opening in April 1975 to August 1976. Omitting 17 deaths and 10 leavers, the final sample consisted of 65 residents (Table 4–1). More than half of the residents were female, as are the majority of persons on the lengthy waiting list.

Description of the Old Age Home Sample

Not all were Catholic, nor were all from Upolu, the island where the home is located, on the outskirts of Apia. In terms of religion, 52 of the 65 were Catholic, 10 Protestant (7 Congregational, 3 Methodist), 2 Mormon and 1 Jewish. Looking at island of origin, 37 were from Upolu and 20 from Savai'i, with three from the Tokelaus and one each from other islands. More than two-fifths thus originated elsewhere.

I attempted to establish the source of referral and reason for admission. Referral sources for eight persons were not known or recorded. Of the remaining 63, 32 were considered self-referred and 29 as referred by families; only two were referred by a hospital or doctor.

Age	Total	Male	Female
60–69	13	9	4
70–79	24	9	15
80–89	23	11	12
90–99	4	1	3
100+	1	0	1
	65	30	35

Source: Little, V. C. _Aging in Western Samoa_, 1976.

TABLE 4–1. Old Age Home Sample

Admissions sometimes included family members, in six cases women to be with ill husbands; a family group of three, including retarded daughter; and another group of two, consisting of mother and disabled daughter. With these exceptions, most admissions were related to medical problems requiring nursing care, or to severe disabilities, or both. Only one was clearly a case of social isolation, and in only four cases was there any evidence of family rejection.

There was a wide range of serious medical conditions, including senility (9 cases), filariasis (8), asthma (5), general debility and weakness of legs (5), arthritis, (5), post-stroke (4), inability to walk (3), cardiac failure (2) and diabetes (2). Other reasons for admission included eye problems, tuberculosis, leprosy, mental illness, mental retardation, central nervous system disorder, cephalgia, vaginitis, and chronic constipation.

The Sisters classify health status according to the New Zealand system: ambulatory, frail or bedfast. On this basis 35 were ambulatory, 19 frail, and 11 bedfast. More of the ambulatory were female, in part because accompanying family members were included. For the frail, the numbers were 10 females and 9 males. Of the 11 bedfast, however, 8 were males.

As reported by nurses, 28 were in "good" health, 32 "fair" and 5 "poor." Those in "poor" health were all males, those in "fair" health were evenly divided, whereas some two-thirds of those in "good" health were female.

Their capacity to see, hear, and walk and the condition of their teeth were also investigated. In this category data were available on 71 patients, including a few leavers. Vision and mobility were the chief problem areas, hearing less so. Of the 23 cases of poor vision, 11 were totally blind and 2 blind in one eye; 3 had cataracts and 7 had other eye problems. One resident was both blind and deaf. As in the community group, many had bad teeth, with 21 characterized as "poor" and 16 as "fair." Only a few had dentures. Whatever their capacity to cut their own toenails, this was done for them by the Sisters.

The Community Sample

The health status and reasons for admission of the institutional sample may be compared with a community sample of 62 persons, interviewed as part of the same project, consisting of 31 males and 31 females (Table 4–2).

Most of those interviewed were members of the centrally located Congregational Christian (London Missionary Society) Church; six were Mormon and two Catholic. There were 39 persons aged 60 and over and 23 between 50 and 60. Of the 62, 49 reported their health as "good" and 12 as "fair"; none reported health as "poor." Eight of the 12 reporting their health to be "fair" were men and four were women.

Sub-Village	M + F	M	F	50-59 M	F	60-69 M	F	70-79 M	F	80-89 M	F	90-99 M	F	100+ M	F
Safua	24	11	13	2	4	6	4	3	3	-	1	-	-	-	1*
Lalomalava	31	18	13	7	6	7	3	4	4	-	-	-	-	-	-
Vaisa'ulu	6	2	4	1	3	1	1	-	-	-	-	-	-	-	-
Vai'afai	1	-	1	x	x	x	x	x	x	x	x	x	x	-	1**
	62	31	31	10	13	14	8	7	7	-	1	-	-	-	2

* age not verified

** age verified

Source: Little, V. C. Aging in Western Samoa, 1976.

TABLE 4–2. The Community Sample

Almost all could perform the activities of daily living (feeding, dressing, bathing, toileting and cutting their toenails) without difficulty; even two of the blind were active, ambulatory and not housebound. In only two cases was help given with toileting and cutting toenails, and in three others with toenails alone.

Seeing difficulties were far more prevalent than hearing ones. A total of 39 reported some difficulty in seeing by comparison with 19 reporting no difficulty; four were blind, two in one eye only. There were three who were deaf, one in one ear only, but only four others reported difficulty with hearing. No one in the community group was unable to walk; however, 32 admitted some problem, which had an important effect on their daily activities, because the plantations were five miles away.

Most persons reported having seen a doctor at least once, usually in connection with surgery or an accident. Only one saw a doctor regularly, every other month. Three had been seen by a doctor or dentist for the purpose of having teeth extracted. Two others were visited at home by the district nurse, but this was considered exceptional. Nine persons had never seen a doctor.

A total of 23 took some pills or medication and nine more reported occasionally taking "Aspro"; one used whiskey, and 29 took no medication at all. Twenty reported having Samoan massage, usually with a coconut oil mixture, done either by relatives or the *fofo*.

When asked, "If you are sick, who takes care of you?", the answer in 47 cases was a member of the immediate family, living in the same *fale*, or nearby: spouse (5), spouse and children (22), daughter (11), children (9). In 12 other cases it would be a member of the extended family: daughter-in-law and son (5), son-in-law (3), sibling (1), "family" (2).

One man reported that his deceased mother (aged 130) would always be there to help him. There was obvious reluctance to go outside the family. In two cases, people said they would call on relatives in another village, or in Apia. Only one said that the women's committee would come when his wife asked; another, who also needed help, preferred notifying relatives from elsewhere, rather than the committee.

The older persons studied had poor teeth, with many missing. Although there is now a dentist in the vicinity, only two reported ever having used his services. Others said they had had teeth extracted at the district hospital, or else they "just dropped out." The oldest respondent, aged 100, said that she pulled out her own when they began to fall out. Only three persons interviewed had dentures. There was one with no teeth, and 13 reporting "poor," or "only a few teeth left." Fifteen reported "fair," with some extracted or falling out. Some 27 said their teeth were "good," with only a few gone.

The condition of teeth bears an obvious relationship to the food usually consumed. Most reported eating all Samoan foods and *palagi* (foreign) foods when available. Those with no or only a few teeth ate mainly soft foods. The person who prepares the food, like the person who cares for you when you are sick, is usually a member of the immediate family, often children and grandchildren, not necessarily female. In only seven cases was it done by "self" or "wife," and in six others by "self and children" or "wife and children."

Over half considered themselves "very active." Except for three reporting "the same" activity as ten years before, the majority described themselves as "less active." Several commented, "I do the same things, but I'm getting slower."

There were five males in the group who reported fishing and farming daily or almost daily and another male, a carpenter, who worked every day. Except for these, and five who reported the women's committee as a major activity, the chief daily pastimes of older people tended to be confined to the *fale* and its immediate surroundings, with occasional trips to the plantation. There was no sharp differentiation between male and female activities. Typical were weaving (mats by women, sennet by men), playing with grandchildren, weeding and cutting grass. Women were more apt to report sweeping and tidying the house or doing laundry. Both sexes reported sitting, talking, eating, and playing cards.

Definition of Old Age

This coincided with the definition of old age which some respondents gave, in answer to the question, "How can you tell when a person is old in Western Samoa?" One answer is "by the way he speaks and acts." The more usual answer is: "A person is old when he finds it hard to get about and do the work he did; so he sits in the house, waits for someone to give food, and tells the family what to do."

Old age, according to a few, is a time of respect: "An old person is given the first and best of everything, even though a *matai* (chief) is there"; or "On special occasions he speaks first and is the most respected." One person described the life cycle as follows: "A baby crawls and is breast-fed; at 10 he starts to work. He has strength until he is 30, between 30 and 40 he has not as much strength. At 50 he has slowed down, and at 60 he stays in the house, waits for food and gives orders."

According to another, being old in Samoa is "a good time of life . . . one sits and waits for people to do the work, unlike Europeans, who save for their old age." According to others, it is both a happy and a sad time. "An old person is happy when his family is happy"; "he is happy because his family takes good care of him; he is sad if someone dies, or if he has differences with other families."

At what age is a person considered old? Here responses varied from "around 30" to "100." The modal answer was aged 50, or more. Some said "around 70" or "when they stop working"; or "70 or 80 is an old person, then they die."

Changing Attitudes Toward Closed Care

In the later interviews respondents were also asked whether they had heard of the new old age home in Apia and, if so, what their opinion was. Only 20 of the persons asked had heard of it and had opinions. Most of the opinions offered reiterated the traditional view that, in Samoa, the family takes care of its old people, who prefer "to stay in their children's hands." "If you go to such a home, it looks as though your children don't love you, or don't want you any more." However, there might be mitigating circumstances such as, "If a family doesn't have enough things to help"; "if there are no children in the home to prepare food"; "if people want to live alone and not hear anything, like bad things about their family's troubles."

Reports of good care in the old age home are widespread, and one person stated " . . . the Bishop [sic] built the home because he loves the old people." However, there was no one from the sub-villages we studied in the home at that time, and most people didn't know anyone there. One opined, "People in Lalomalava are stronger than in Apia." One old person interviewed said that he wouldn't mind going to the home and might apply, after his sons came home from New Zealand in October for a family conference; he thought he would prefer it to migrating to New Zealand, where the climate is too cold.

Comparison of the Community and Institutional Samples

Because persons in their fifties were included in the community sample, the age distribution of the two groups is not comparable. The institutional group was drawn from various places on the two main islands and elsewhere, and reflected in part the admissions policies of the old age home. The community group had only three persons aged 80 and over, all female, whereas persons in their seventies and eighties predominated in the institutional group, which also had five persons aged 90 and over.

The institutional group was not only older, but more female. It was also more incapacitated. Whereas no persons in the community were bedfast, only three were housebound, and no one was unable to walk, the institution had 11 bedfast patients, and 19 frail, including many wheelchair cases. However, there is no sharp dividing line by which persons in a home are handicapped, whereas those in the community are not; the home had 35 ambulatory patients, compared with 33 in the community reporting some difficulty in walking, often using a stick.

Index of Incapacity

A simple index of incapacity was calculated for each person, based on eight items: see, hear, walk, feed, dress, bathe, toilet, and toenails. A person having no difficulty with the activity was scored 0; those unable to perform or experiencing difficulty were scored 1. A total score of 0 thus indicates no incapacity; a score of 8 maximum incapacity. Scores of 0–2 were ranked as minimal incapacity, 3–5 somewhat incapacitated, and 6–8 severely incapacitated (Table 4–3).

The community group had no severely incapacitated persons and only six who were moderately so, by comparison with 56 who were minimally incapacitated, including nine who had no stated incapacities. By contrast, the institutional group had 15 severely incapacitated and 22 who were moderately so. A total of 28, half as many as in the community, had minimal incapacity.

According to age, the six most incapacitated persons in the community ranged from 54 to 100; two were in their fifties, one in the sixties, two in the

Score	Community			Institution		
	M + F	M	F	M + F	M	F
Minimal						
0	9	4	5	–	–	–
1	30	15	15	18	8	10
2	17	9	8	10	5	5
Subtotal	56	28	28	28	13	15
Somewhat						
3	5	3	2	14	6	8
4	–	–	–	5	3	2
5	1	–	1	3	2	1
Subtotal	6	3	3	22	11	11
Severely						
6	–	–	–	2	1	1
7	–	–	–	8	3	5
8	–	–	–	5	2	3
Subtotal	–	–	–	15	6	9
Total	62	31	31	65	30	35

Source: Little, V. C. Aging in Western Samoa, 1976.

TABLE 4–3. Index of Incapacity, Community and Institutional Groups, by Sex

seventies and one a possible 100. Three were male and three female. The 15 most incapacitated old age home residents ranged in age from 65 to a reported 104; they were scattered over the entire age range, with seven in their eighties. Six were male and nine female.

Summary

The issue of open or closed care is thus fairly joined in Western Samoa, a traditional society in the process of transition. That families care for their old people is still true in the villages studied in rural Savai'i; however, these villages have few severely ill people and few in the older age cohorts receiving care in the Home, which is demonstrating the existence of otherwise unmet needs.

Many questions remain about the ways in which changes in a traditional culture affect aging individuals. Behind the family is an informal support system of women's and church committees which are available for backup but seldom utilized. If out-migration of younger, economically active persons continues, and the extended family structure is further eroded, will this informal sector be utilized more frequently? At present it appears to serve more as an outlet for energetic and able women, and as a system of social control, rather than social services.

Conflicting attitudes toward aging are expressed, sometimes by the same individual. Although the traditional value of family care is always affirmed, the thoughtful point out that some families do a poor job of caring, leaving their old people in leaky, dirty *fales*, and feeding them poorly. A member of the executive committee for the old age home said, "I wouldn't put my mother in the home, but I have brought four of my old 'uncles' and 'aunties' here; one didn't like it, so we took him home again."

It is still considered important to die and be buried at home with proper ceremonies; one informant stated that this is partly because there are seldom written wills and the last wishes of the dying need to be heard by the family. For whatever reasons, some dying residents have insisted on leaving the old age home and have done so; others have died there and their mourners have come to the mortuary for the ceremonies.

My own view is related to my overall hypotheses that the number of institutions for the old is increasing in every country and that the level of investment in closed care tends to exceed that in open care, at every stage of economic and social development. I would predict that, in Western Samoa, as elsewhere, the first old-age home will be followed by others, at first under private and later under public auspices. The informal sector will continue to be available as a backup to the family system. Hopefully, the Samoan ability to harmonize conflict and to tolerate ambiguity will help to cushion the next transition, when the extended family structure no longer suffices.

5

The Hong Kong Experience: Level 2

The experience of Hong Kong, a unique political system, suggests lessons for others, both positive and negative, as well as for its own development. Hong Kong may be viewed as a microcosm, which mirrors in a relatively small area, and within a relatively short time frame, some of the economic, social, and value changes which are having an impact upon care systems in every society.

Background

Before 1945 social welfare policies and programs in the Crown Colony of Hong Kong were little developed. British colonial policy tended to be pragmatic,and remedial, reflecting a Poor Law philosophy which aimed to return the undeserving poor to their countries of origin, and at keeping the colony from serving as a Mecca for poor Chinese and the poor of other Asiatic countries. The Second World War and the Chinese Revolution initiated a change process and forced a new focus on social welfare problems, including those of old people.

The most striking change has been a sizable growth in the total population, from 0.6 million to 4.7 million. This has been accompanied by increasing numbers of elderly, who are now a larger proportion of the total (Figure 5–1). At the end of 1978 there were in Hong Kong 424,000 persons aged 60 and over, amounting to 9.24 percent of the total population, an increase of 23 percent in the decade 1968 to 1978 (Hong Kong, 1979). According to the government's population projections, there will be some 490,000 old people by 1981 and 598,000 by 1986, by then 11.6 percent of the total (Figure 5–2).

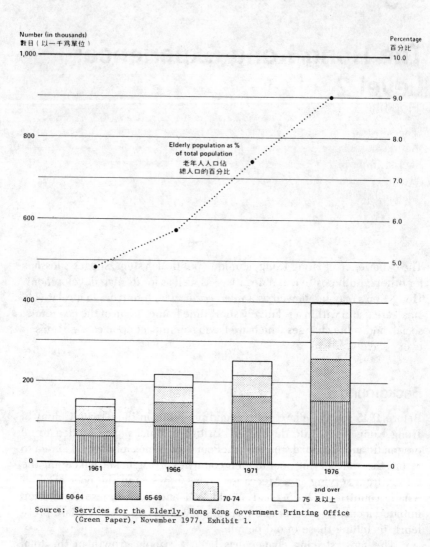

FIGURE 5–1. Age Structure and Size of the Elderly Population of Hong Kong, 1961–1976

Many of the present old came as refugees from mainland China before and after 1949. The flood of immigration, both legal and illegal, is now at the rate of more than 100,000 annually. Some are already old. It is difficult to estimate how many more will be coming from China and from other Southeast Asian countries, and what proportion will be old. New boatloads arrive daily.

At a time when the total population is swelling in an unpredictable and uncontrollable way, what has been the societal response to past and projected increases in its elder population?

Housing

The most visible part of the response has been to build, and to plan to build, more high-rise housing estates not only on Hong Kong Island but increasingly in the New Territories, where three new towns are being created (Tsuen Wan, Tuen Mun, Sha Tin), each with a large component of planned public housing, to be supplemented by private. It is estimated that 45 percent of the population now lives in public housing.

This substantial housing effort has reduced, but not eliminated, squatter and shanty settlements, street sleepers, boat people and waiting lists. One reason that the new wave of migration is so threatening is that it jeopardizes the precarious equilibrium attained by efforts to date. In particular, it threatens the living situation of the old who, as elsewhere, tend to occupy the least desirable housing. Many rent a bed-space and others linger in hospitals because of lack of accommodation, with family or elsewhere.

One innovation is noteworthy. This is the Hong Kong practice of including so-called "hostels" for the elderly in the more recently built estates. These consist of a floor or floors set aside for them; special personal care units for those who become frail are found in some. Hostels have been helpful to those admitted. By and large, however, the old have suffered from space provisions and regulations favoring nuclear families; for example, until recently, a unit could not be shared by three unrelated adults. The marginal situation of poor single older men, some of whom live in so-called "cages," has produced newspaper publicity, but to date little official action.

Health/Medical

Hong Kong lacks a health insurance scheme, and so far has made no special provision for the medical and health needs of the elderly as a categorical group. The health/medical system in the colony reflects both British standards and overseas training and traditional Chinese medicine. The University of Hong Kong has a medical school, and the Chinese University is planning to start one within two years. There are local nursing programs, but severe shortages of technicians, in particular physical and occupational therapists.

The medical sector is more developed than the social services sector,

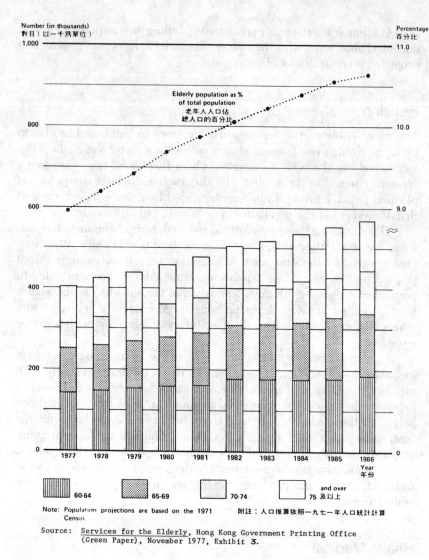

Source: Services for the Elderly, Hong Kong Government Printing Office
(Green Paper), November 1977, Exhibit 3.

FIGURE 5–2. Projection of the Elderly Population of Hong Kong, 1977–1986

and has both a group of designated regional hospitals and a ten-year
medical development plan. Persons of all ages may utilize government
clinics at the nominal price of $1 HK for each visit; medication is also
supplied. However, the level of availability, acceptability and accessibility
is considerably below the apparent need of the population at risk.

The problem of shortfall bears especially on the frail elderly, who, if they seek help, must arise early, arrange their own transportation, and often sit all day in a clinic without being seen by medical personnel. For understandable reasons the elderly patient often prefers traditional Chinese herbal remedies and procedures such as acupuncture.

A model geriatrics program and day hospital is located at Princess Margaret Hospital; others are being started, for example, health education is beginning in Caritas Medical Centre, mainly in the form of public exhibits of slides and photographs, and a small-group approach is underway at United Christian Hospital. The old are included, but programs are aimed mainly at younger subjects.

The possibility of a health scheme for the elderly that is comparable to that for schoolchildren has been temporarily shelved by the government. There is little or no medical care in most of the 23 old-age homes which have been studied by the Hong Kong Council of Social Service; in fact, a resident is less likely to have seen a doctor in the past year than an old person in the community (Hong Kong Council of Social Service Needs Study, 1978).

Income Maintenance

In Hong Kong the more generic term "social security" is used to cover all forms of income maintenance. Although civil servants are pensioned, there is no contributory system of social insurance for most workers and few private pensions. Since 1971 there has been a public assistance scheme, and since 1973 a demogrant, now called an "old age allowance," of $100 HK monthly. In response to public pressure the age of eligibility was lowered from 75 to 70 as of October 1978. By April 1, 1979 this had resulted in an additional caseload of 65,000 old people, with an even larger number of applicants waiting to be processed.

For the elderly poor various supplements and "improvements," introduced in April 1978, are available to augment the meager public assistance allowance. As in Britain, these may have the effect of obscuring the "single safety net" principle, without necessarily increasing benefits significantly (Chow, 1978). Under present policy the old age allowance is also paid to residents of institutions, who are expected to use it for their medical, clothing, and other expenses, as well as for pocket money.

In terms of number of recipients and impact on the population at risk, the program of financial payments is the largest single program. The ingenuity of paying old people an allowance and then in turn requiring them to pay for services would be deplored in more developed welfare states, but may appeal to developing countries striving to stave off social insurance and to keep welfare payments low.

The Planning and Policy Framework

For both developed and developing countries, what Alvin Schorr once termed "paper planning" prevails. Especially where elderservices are concerned, rhetoric exceeds resource allocation, in particular for open care.

Here, too, Hong Kong offers the ingredients for a useful case study. There have been two waves of official policy statements, one in 1973 and again in 1977–1979 (Government Printer, Hong Kong). The first consisted of three separate documents and was centered around "The Five-Year Plan for Social Welfare Development in Hong Kong, 1973–78," then considered a model and reflecting a new kind of joint partnership between the public and private sectors. The plan was based on a major policy statement, "Social Welfare in Hong Kong: The Way Ahead," which replaced an earlier and more limited paper dated May, 1965. The third of the triad, "Care in the Community: The Right Basis for Services to the Elderly," was the report of a Working Party on the Future Needs of the Elderly; this recommended pushing ahead to establish a satisfactory framework early, while resource costs were still comparatively low. Unfortunately, this viewpoint did not prevail.

The second wave of policy statements, that of 1977–1979, included separate documents on children and youth, on integrating the disabled into the community, and on social security development. The most controversial of the second group turned out to be the Green Paper on Services for the Elderly, issued in November 1977, which failed to turn white until April 1979, when a paper entitled "Social Welfare into the 1980's" was issued (Government Printer, Hong Kong).

The White Paper of April, 1979

The government's present stance has not changed greatly since 1973. It is essentially a vulnerable groups strategy aimed at the poor, the elderly, and the disabled. This means continuing rejection of a universal strategy with minimum guarantees or entitlements for all. It also means that the government reserves the right of decision on labelling additional groups as vulnerable. For example, the 1979 paper favors putting the "profoundly deaf" under the disability allowance, but rejects "chronic sickness" and "moderate mental retardation" as categories to be added. In principle, all persons should be encouraged to work, although some uncertainty is felt about the chronically ill between 60 and 70 years of age.

In terms of target groups, the disabled are listed first, followed by the elderly, followed by young people. This is a partial resolution of the young versus the old dilemma, which the 1973 working party had characterized as a value choice to be made by the community. Has the community in fact decided that the old now have a higher priority than the young? Why have the disabled been advanced to a preferred category?

Occupational benefits and sickness, injury and death benefit schemes appear to have low priority and are deferred as needing further study and consideration. A cautious governmental attitude is also apparent in adding to social welfare services. The White Paper states that services for the elderly are to be expanded "on a wide front," with a three-fold strategy of improving cash benefits, providing more institutional beds, and "promoting social integration of the elderly within the community." Where are open care and services like home help and day care? Apparently the principal service will continue to be financial, in the form of the old age allowance, seen not only as promoting independent living, but also as an incentive to encourage families to look after their elderly members (Government Printer, Hong Kong).

Impact of Planning on Services, 1973–1978

Overall, the 1979 White Paper suggests a subtle shift of emphasis since 1973, when the planning objective was stated as: "To assist the elderly to remain in the community at large, while expanding and improving residential care 'to the extent necessary.' " In fact, the stated objective was not reflected in the first five-year plan, which gave top priority to closed care, and proposed no extension of open care until the fifth year.

Planning and implementation do not always proceed at the same rate. Recognizing this, the government has instituted a new planning review procedure, again with the participation of the voluntary sector. This is a somewhat cumbersome process, which requires some 18 months lead time. This delay, however, acts as a device for picking up changing priorities as well as difficulties in implementing the plan for the previous year.

Few data on implementation are available. What is known suggests that the record is a spotty one, due in part to changes in the overall economic climate and budgetary constraints and in part to delays in obtaining land, approval, and funding for new building projects. A particular problem has been to significantly increase the number of "care and attention" (chronic) beds, still in very short supply. Meanwhile, services to maintain old people in open care, such as community nursing and home help, have had to fight for their place in the budget; with major funding constraints, they are weakly developed.

As of October 31, 1978 there were in existence seven hostels for the elderly, with a total capacity of 696; 22 subvented old age homes, with a capacity of 2,627; three care and attention homes, with a capacity of 233;

one multi-service center; and 16 social centers. Four agencies were de-livering some form of home help service and a total of nine were engaged in community nursing.

The 1979 White Paper, like the previous one, is to be read in conjunc-tion with the current five-year plan. For the planning periods 1978–1979 and 1985–1986 planned projects include ten hostels, six home help ser-vices, five multi-service centers, three day care centers, 17 social centers, 16 homes for the aged and 13 care and attention homes. The major planned expansion of open care services is for community nursing, not subsidized earlier and now to be 100 percent subvented, with plans to train 300 additional nurses over the next five-year period. The planned expansion of home helpers is considerably lower, from 40 to 55 in the first year, with an additional 40 helpers annually thereafter.

The White Paper speaks of two "experimental" day care centers, each catering to 80 people, to be operated by the voluntary sector. However, by 1982–1983 the government plans to provide an additional 117 "social" centers for the elderly, and eventually to achieve a ratio of one center for every 20,000 of the population. Family life education is approved, under the aegis of the Urban Council, along with the bulk booking of tickets for recreational events.

Counseling and visiting services are encouraged, but on a voluntary basis. A new thrust is the statement that community services should be coordinated on a "district" basis, presumably a reference to the Social Welfare Department's regionalization plan. To date, the voluntary sector, which supplies all of the services, has not been regionalized. The official goal, however, is 17 "multi-service" centers, one for each district, of which seven are to be begun in 1980–1981. People aged 55 and over are encour-aged to work and to retire flexibly, with plans for two trial part-time handicraft centers by the 1980–1981 year (Government Printing, 16–17).

Gap Between Planning Goals and Need Levels

The policy response of the government appears on examination to be a constrained one, with limited subsidization of open care. That govern-ment's planning goals fall considerably below the known needs level has been documented by a joint Hong Kong Council of Social Service/Social Welfare Department survey. An even greater gap is seen when one examines actual service delivery levels. Figures previously published in the *Welfare Digest* document this point (Table 5–2). Tables 5–1 and 5–2 underline not only the gaps in planning and service delivery, but also reinforce the point that the principal service for old people in Hong Kong is

Type of Service	Percent of Those 60+ in Need	Estimated Number Persons in Need	Planned Green Paper Provisions
Hostel	6.06%	37,590	5,000 places
Home for the Elderly	2.32%	14,390	4,962 places
Care and Attention Home	0.4%	2,481	2,481
Geriatric Hospital	1.29%	5,401*	1,077 beds
Home Help Service	2.32%	14,390	310 helpers
Community Nursing	2.49%	15,197	210 nurses
Public Housing	5.94%	30,704	5,000 places

*for those aged 65+

Source: Adapted from Welfare Digest, Issue No. 60, p. 3. Additional data for needs study. By courtesy of Welfare Digest (official publication of The Hong Kong Council of Social Service, Hong Kong).

TABLE 5–1. Planned Provisions for the Elderly Population of Hong Kong by the Year 1987, in relation to the Percentages and Numbers of Persons with Such Needs

cash payments. By comparison, the numbers receiving any other service is very small. Less than one percent of the population at risk is institutionalized; this might be considered a positive indicator if more community services were in fact available. However, a rough calculation indicates that less than one-tenth of one percent participate in community services of any kind.

Mix of Open, Closed, and Unorganized Care

Additional data may be drawn from the Hong Kong Council's needs study, previously cited. According to this, a similar population of frail, aging illiterate females is found in all three kinds of care. Only a very small percentage has access to the formal system.

In fact, the majority lack information on the existence of services, including social clubs. Where do old people living in Hong Kong turn when in need of help? Most consult family members and relatives, with neighbors and friends listed as second. Only 1.36 percent had ever talked to professionals and outsiders such as social workers, priests or church members. Some eight percent had nobody with whom to consult. Over

Type of Service	Number of Agencies/Centers	Number of Recipients
1. Transit Centers	1	28
2. Hostels		510
3. Old People's Homes	19	2,740
4. Old People's Homes (for the blind)	2	104
5. Care and Attention Homes	2	116
6. Geriatric Units	3	164
7. Home Help	3	95
8. Community Nursing	9	989*
9. Meals	2	229
10. Employment Service	1	15
11. Sheltered Workshop	1	–
12. Old People's Clubs	40	5,000
13. Regional Federations	5	–
14. Public Assistance	1	29,747**
15. Infirmity Allowance	1	52,281***

    * Between 1973 & 1975
  ** Up to May 1976
*** Up to March 1976

Source: Welfare Digest, Issue No. 41, p. 5. By courtesy of Welfare Digest (official publication of The Hong Kong Council of Social Service, Hong Kong).

TABLE 5–2. Services for the Elderly Population of Hong Kong, January 1977

three-fourths had never heard of old people's clubs, and another 18 percent had heard of them but did not know their function. It is no surprise that 95 percent had never participated.

The most disadvantaged groups appear to be those in closed care. They tend to have a higher median age, a higher female/male ratio and a slightly higher illiteracy rate than those still living in the community. An interesting difference is that more than 70 percent in closed care are worshippers of formal religions, compared with less than 20 percent of the community sample. Almost two-thirds had lived alone before moving into residential care; a total of 78 percent had no family members living in Hong Kong.

The study contains abundant data that the residential group receives little or no care in many of the settings studied. Although more frail, they are less likely to receive medical care and attention. A majority of the homes are understaffed, and residents often do their own cooking and laundry as well as personal care. In part due to less than ideal conditions, there is a very high vacancy rate in existing homes, 436 places or 13.4 percent of the total. The Council's overall finding is even more striking: more than 70 percent of old people are presently placed at inappropriate levels of care (Hong Kong Council, Needs Study, pp. 42–79).

The findings on the residential sample also suggest gaps in the unorganized care sector. The majority enter residential care because they lack

family supports. A minority have relatives but have poor family relationships, with little respect and little likelihood that occasions such as
their birthdays will be remembered. Hong Kong social workers face daily
the necessity of finding a bed-space for an older person left in the hospital
with no place to go. Is the answer an old age allowance which is the
equivalent of about United States $20 monthly?

Summing Up

The dilemma of Hong Kong is the dilemma of many societies: deficits in all
three care systems. The task of simultaneously upgrading closed care,
building a network of open care, and shoring up unorganized care is one
which strains the existing level of resource allocation, and seems to require
major changes in approach and philosophy. What is the place of aging
cohorts, some refugees, in an urban Oriental setting? What proportion of
known needs should be met by public provision?

Looking back over the road recently travelled in a search for the way
ahead, what are some of the gains, potential gains and negatives, as seen by
an outside observer?

The major gains would include:

1. Institution of a means-tested public assistance scheme;
2. Institution of a disability and infirmity allowance (now renamed
"old age allowance"), in effect a demogrant, and lowering of the age of
eligibility from 75 to 70;
3. Provision of special hostels or floors for old people, as part of public
housing estates;
4. The policy decision to subvent community nursing, and to increase subsidies for home help and related services;
5. Beginnings of support for day care for the elderly;
6. Some subsidization of new old age homes, especially care and
attention homes;
7. A model geriatric program in Princess Margaret Hospital, including a day hospital, and the setting aside of geriatric beds in other hospitals;
8. Beginnings of health education of the elderly and inclusion of the
elderly in family life education;
9. A major research study of the social service needs of the elderly
completed by the Hong Kong Council of Social Service in March 1978 and
other studies in progress;
10. Hosting of three major international social welfare conferences in
the summer of 1980.

More problematic, but potentially positive are:

1. Regionalization of the Social Welfare Department into defined districts, to be followed by possible regionalization of the voluntary sector;
2. Encouragement for more "multi-service" and "social" centers for the old;
3. A continuing working arrangement between the public and private sectors to fund and deliver community services;
4. Concern over the quality of care in institutions, and beginning attempts to improve this by manipulating the rate of subvention.

I see the following as essentially negative, that is if the goal is "to reach the whole of each client group as soon as possible":

1. Ambivalence over the traditional Chinese family system, in the face of mounting evidence that this has been eroded in modern, urban, industrial Hong Kong;
2. Continuing reliance on an outmoded 19th-century model of voluntarism to meet major needs;
3. The downgrading of professional social work skills and contributions;
4. Low levels of public assistance and old age allowances, linked to the dubious principle that these can somehow be used to have old people pay for their own services;
5. Disregard of available research data, especially that on needs;
6. Poor governmental structure in the composition of the Social Welfare Advisory Committee, and time-consuming procedures in planning and budgeting.

The negatives just listed essentially reflect elevation of the goal of cost containment to center stage as the "real" objective of service programs along with the accumulation of budgetary surpluses, for which high social costs are paid in the living levels of vulnerable groups, such as the old and the poor. Hong Kong, like other societies, still has miles to go in closing the gap between the two faces of care, that which is available on paper, and that which is available in fact.

6

Japan as an Example
of Level 3

Japan has been chosen as an example of Level 3: rapid transition and expansion from a public welfare base. It is a little-studied case of the development of a modern welfare system which, since 1963, has placed increasing emphasis on services for old people.

In thinking about Japan, as about Western Samoa, there is a tendency for myths and leading images to prevail over facts. Japan is simultaneously admired by less developed countries as an industrialized success story that retained traditional values of filial piety and the Confucian ethic, and by Western Japanologists as having preserved the status of "the honorable elders" more successfully than other developed societies (Palmore, 1975). Another recent work by a well-known American scholar is titled "Japan as Number One" and refers to Japan's leading position in social welfare, basic education, crime control, and other key areas (Vogel, 1979).

Other experts suggest that traditional Japanese society, as characterized by Benedict in the felicitous phrase "the chrysanthemum and the sword," is changing, just as other societies are changing. This rate of change has accelerated since 1945. Thus, some scholars find in Japan evidence of considerable ambivalence toward the old. They point to the high rate of elderly suicide, especially for aging females, and find that there are equally powerful negative images, such as the Obasute tradition and "the hateful age" (Plath, 1972).

Japan demonstrated its leadership in gerontology by hosting the XIth International Congress in Tokyo in August 1978. At the Congress and since the Japanese have shown deep concern over the changing age structure of their population (Table 6–1). As they see it, Japan, which achieved an "aged" age structure only in 1970, is advancing more rapidly than have other industrialized nations into the "era of man-made longevity." Looking at official population projections (Table 6–2), they worry about the increasing number and proportion of dependent older people.

The Japanese are far from satisfied with their present services, even though they have grown, and are assiduously adding programs and seeking new approaches and answers. They are also keenly aware of the changing

Year	Percent Distribution by Age Group		
	0 – 14 Years Old	15 – 64 Years Old	65 Years Old and Over
1920	36.48	58.26	5.26
1925	36.70	58.24	5.06
1930	36.59	58.66	4.75
1935	36.89	58.46	4.66
1940	36.08	59.19	4.43
1947	35.30	59.90	4.79
1950	35.37	59.69	4.94
1955	33.38	61.30	5.32
1960	30.04	64.23	5.73
1965	25.61	68.10	6.29
1970	23.93	69.00	7.07
1975	24.32	67.72	7.92

Source: Census results. The population of Okinawa Perfecture is included in those in 1975 and before 1940.

TABLE 6–1. Change of Age Structure of the Japanese Population, 1920–1975

Year	Percent Distribution of Age Group		
	0 – 14 Years Old	15 – 64 Years Old	65 Years Old and Over
1975	24.29	67.76	7.91
1980	24.01	67.11	8.88
1985	22.90	67.36	9.74
1990	20.97	68.01	11.01
1995	20.10	67.21	12.69
2000	20.16	65.58	14.26
2005	20.51	64.04	15.45
2010	20.27	63.00	16.72
2015	19.56	61.90	18.54
2020	19.15	62.04	18.81
2025	19.35	62.54	18.12
2030	19.84	62.60	17.56
2035	19.99	62.57	17.44
2040	19.70	62.33	17.97
2045	19.37	62.40	18.23
2050	19.39	62.51	18.10

Source: Future Population Projections for Japan as projected in November 1976, Institute of Population Problems, Ministry of Health and Welfare, Tokyo, November 1976.

TABLE 6–2. Future Age Structure of Japanese Population, 1975–2050

values and mores which are having an impact on work and retirement practices, the co-residence of aged parents with adult offspring, and other aspects of the living situation of the old.

Background

Before the Second World War, a rapidly industrializing Japan relied largely on the semi-feudalistic family system to absorb the tensions and strains of economic and social change. The first step toward social insurance was not taken until 1922, in the form of limited health insurance. There was no national system of retirement insurance until 1942 (Shimada in Dessau, 1968).

The loss of the war and the adoption of the MacArthur constitution brought an influx of American advisers, including social welfare experts and professional social workers. In the early postwar years livelihood protection, workmen's compensation and unemployment insurance laws were passed, followed by more comprehensive social insurance and assistance legislation. The present framework of income maintenance, public pensions, and medical insurance dates from 1973.

The early postwar years were focused on developing programs for children and youth. Beginning in the 1960s, however, growing awareness of the changing population structure sparked interest in services for old people.

Law for the Welfare of the Aged, 1963

The basic law for the welfare of the aged was passed in July 1963. Its affirmation of a mutuality of obligations between the older members and society is frequently cited with approval, although it may not be juridically binding (Broberg et al., 1975). The key article is Article 4, by which the Central Government and local public body "have the responsibility to promote the welfare of the aged." The law then goes on to assign specific functions to Social Welfare Secretaries, the Welfare Office, the Health Center, and Welfare Visitors, at the prefectural, city, town, and village levels.

An annual health examination is provided, and September 15 designated as Old People's Day. It is the responsibility of local government to place persons "not less than 65 years" under guidance, and sometimes guardianship; in nursing homes, special nursing homes or foster homes; to arrange funerals as required; and to send home helpers to take care of the aged in their own homes when, "owing to physical or mental breakdown, they . . . have trouble with the conduct of daily life." Health promotion, cultural and recreational activities are also mentioned, along with assistance to Old People's Clubs and "other persons promoting the welfare of the aged."

This broad mandate represents a policy decision to follow the example of advanced welfare states, such as Sweden and Britain, in adopting a public welfare model that places responsibility for service delivery at the local government level. Before passing their own law, the Japanese had studied the experiences of other countries and had experimented with services on a small scale. From the first there was a focus on home help as the core service for open care around which other supplementary services may cluster. This too copies overseas practice.

How Home Help Started; How It Grew

Home help was first introduced in Japan in 1955, in Ueda City, by a local welfare officer who had observed it in England. The next year a second service was started in Nagana prefecture by a Japanese who had been in the United States. However, it is the British model which has predominated, along with the English name "home help" (Little, 1975a).

The decade 1965–1975 was marked by a notable growth of home help services under public auspices (Table 6–3). Growth has continued since 1975, although there is an apparent leveling of effort in the total number of helpers reported as working with the aged: *viz.*, 9,220 in May 1973; 8,706 in December 1976; 9,213 in September 1978.

Between 1975 and 1978 there has been a continuing increase in the total number of households served, as well as the numbers of households with old people. Strict eligibility requirements limit the receipt of services to those households not required to pay income tax in Japan. Of the households served in 1978, 36.1 percent of those served by helpers for the aged were on public assistance, by comparison with 26.2 percent of those served by others (Table 6–4).

The Three-tiered System

The public welfare sector is only one of the sources of home help services in Japan. At present there is a three-tiered system, with each tier aimed at different target populations: (1) *public welfare* for the aged, the disabled, crippled children, and some low-income families; (2) *industrial* for the households of persons employed in certain industries, including the executives, white- and blue-collar workers; and (3) *proprietary* for those who can

Year	Total	Having Home Help		Management Helpers			Public Assist.	Others	Only O.P. 60+	Incl'g O.P. 60+
		No.	%	Trust No.	Employed	Total				
1965	3,375	229	6.8	-	673	6,890	5,768	1,122	6,062	828
1966	3,352	316	9.4	138	855	7,399	6,212	1,187	6,633	766
1967	3,303	451	13.7	202	1,108	9,608	7,624	1,884	8,596	912
1968	3,298	638	19.3	291	1,338	13,877	10,927	2,950	12,584	1,293
1969	3,284	1,960	59.7	804	4,145	25,785	14,164	11,621	19,256	6,529
1970	3,257	2,223	68.3	806	4,746	30,801	15,790	15,011	22,636	8,165
1971	3,237	2,533	78.3	1,045	5,586	37,586	17,769	19,817	28,069	9,517
1972	3,277	2,769	84.5	1,022	6,298	45,104	20,763	24,341	33,794	11,310
1973	3,277	2,940	89.7	1,070	7,278	53,140	22,674	30,466	39,686	13,454
1974*	3,267	2,950	90.3	1,087	7,657	56,454	24,012	32,442	42,383	14,071

*First 6 months only

Source: Prime Minister's Office, Japan. Statistics on programs for the aged, September 1975.

TABLE 6–3. Growth of Home Help Services in Japan, 1965–1975

Number	Total	Management Trust
1. Number of cities & towns having home help services	3,175	1,226
2. Number of home helpers		
(a) for the aged	9,213	3,550
(b) for others	2,211	788
	11,424	4,338
3. Number of households served		
(a) only O.P. 604	51,086	–
(b) encl. G.O.P. 604	15,876	–
(c) others	13,871	–
	80,833	–

Source: Data supplied by Mr. Y. Shimizu, Tokyo Metropolitan Institute of Gerontology.

TABLE 6–4. Level of Home Help Service in Japan as of September 30, 1978

pay the charges, or are otherwise covered by disability or workmen's compensation insurance.

The expansion of services has required more workers in all three sectors. However, data are lacking for those not falling under the jurisdiction of the Ministry of Health and Welfare. The industrial sector is said to be small, with about 450 helpers employed by some 350 firms. The number of persons employed in the proprietary sector is variously reported as anywhere from 67,000 to 120,000 registrants, not all of whom may be active at any given time.

The Cross-national Project

In 1975 10 American scholars, of whom I was one, were selected by the U.S. Gerontological Society to work with Japanese colleagues on research projects of mutual concern. The one reported here is entitled "A Comparison and Evaluation of the Impact and Effect of Home Help Services in Japan and Homemaker-Home Health Aide Services in the United States." Two Japanese research teams were involved: a Ministry of Health and Welfare team, initially under the leadership of Mr. Mikio Mori and later under Mr. Soji Tanaka; and a Tokyo Metropolitan Institute of Gerontology team under the leadership of Mr. Daisaku Maeda (Little, 1978).

The intial research design set the goal of completing 150 recipient interviews in each country, 50 each in a metropolitan area, an adjacent suburban area or "bedroom community," and a nearby rural area. Because of the location of the researchers, the Japanese metropolitan area chosen was Tokyo and vicinity.

Selection of the final samples posed numerous difficulties and led to departures from the original design. For example, in Japan, the city of Kamagawa was selected rather than Suwa, as first planned, resulting in a shrinkage of available recipient cases. The refusal rate was also higher than expected. As a result, the two Japanese teams completed a total of 94 interviews, including 40 in Tokyo, 34 in a Tokyo suburb, and 20 in a rural area on the other side of Tokyo Bay.

The second Japanese team, that of the TMIG, went on to collect additional data about the difficulties of families living with and caring for impaired old people and the characteristics of nonrecipients as well as recipients. Nonrecipients were selected from a larger panel of 4,800 old persons drawn earlier for a study of the need for day care. In all, 408 impaired cases were identified by a mail screening test and follow-up interviews. Using two criteria, family type and capacity to perform the activities of daily living, a sample of 78 cases was selected as those most in need of home help services, 64 of whom were interviewed.

The two groups were not equally matched. In fact, the nonrecipient group was found to have a higher proportion of severely impaired old people (Table 6–5). Among recipients, the aged living alone accounted for 68 percent and aging couples living alone for an additional 15 percent; by contrast, 60 percent of the nonrecipients lived with children. Recipients were 80 percent below Y 100,000 in monthly income; nonrecipients only 25 percent (Honma et al., 1978).

Unmet Needs

Both recipients and nonrecipients have significant unmet needs. In a series of interesting calculations, the Japanese team came up with a "care-need" score and a "housekeeping-need" score. These measures are being refined but the initial results are striking: about 30 percent of nonrecipients are totally and severely impaired. There is also a higher proportion of moderately impaired persons among nonrecipients, whereas three-fifths of the recipients are found to be only mildly impaired and fairly active.

For recipients, who are typically visited twice weekly for two hours each visit, many housekeeping tasks are not being done. Both recipient and nonrecipient households have major unmet needs for additional basic services, such as bathing, Meals on Wheels, home nursing, etc. (Honma et al., 1978).

The assumption that the needs of impaired old people living with adult children are being adequately met by the unorganized care sector is

Incapacitating Condition		Normal		Slightly Impaired		Severely Impaired		Total Impaired	
		Number	%	Number	%	Number	%	Number	%
Sight	Recipient	46	(48.6)	34	(36.2)	9	(9.6)	5	(5.3)
	Nonrecipient	40	(62.6)	18	(28.1)	5	(7.8)	1	(1.6)
Hearing	Recipient	58	(61.7)	29	(30.9)	7	(7.4)	–	–
	Nonrecipient	37	(57.8)	20	(31.3)	7	(10.9)	–	–
Speaking	Recipient	77	(81.9)	13	(13.8)	4	(4.3)	–	–
	Nonrecipient	49	(76.6)	10	(15.6)	2	(3.1)	3	(4.7)
Walking	Recipient	64	(68.1)	21	(22.3)	3	(3.2)	6	(6.4)
	Nonrecipient	37	(57.8)	18	(28.1)	2	(3.1)	7	(10.9)
Dressing	Recipient	50	(53.2)	33	(35.1)	6	(6.4)	5	(5.3)
	Nonrecipient	31	(48.4)	13	(20.3)	10	(15.6)	10	(15.6)
Eating	Recipient	73	(77.7)	13	(13.8)	5	(5.3)	3	(3.2)
	Nonrecipient	41	(64.1)	14	(21.9)	3	(4.7)	6	(9.4)
Control of Bladder*	Recipient	18/30	(60.0)	6/30	(20.0)	2/30	(6.7)	4/30	(13.3)
	Nonrecipient	40/56	(71.4)	8/56	(14.3)	2/56	(3.6)	6/56	(10.7)
Control of Bowels*	Recipient	14/30	(46.7)	9/30	(30.0)	2/30	(6.7)	4/30	(13.3)
	Nonrecipient	45/56	(80.4)	3/56	(5.4)	2/56	(3.6)	6/56	(10.7)
Bathing	Recipient	64	(68.1)	9	(9.6)	5	(5.3)	3	(3.2)
	Nonrecipient	29	(45.3)	10	(15.6)	12	(18.8)	13	(20.3)

*Excluding those who live alone

Source: Summary of Japanese data supplied by D. Maeda, Tokyo Metropolitan Institute of Gerontology, July 15, 1978.

TABLE 6–5. Number and Percent of Japanese Recipients and Nonrecipients of Home Help Services, by Incapacitating Condition and Degree of Impairment, 1977

also questioned by the Japanese team, which analyzed 312 such cases. There is an important distinction between two types of families: "those living with an unmarried child" (58 in number) and "those living with a married child" (254 in number). The first was found to have a higher proportion of severely impaired old people and to be less capable of giving care, in particular when the unmarried child is employed full time. In more than two-thirds of the cases where the primary caretaker was fully employed, there was no subcaretaker. Other relatives, typically married daughters, were able to visit the impaired elderly only once weekly or less. In these situations the frail old people had to rely mainly on self-care (Shimizu et al., 1978).

Meanwhile, caretaking families reported major difficulties, such as being tired, poor household management, problems with the family business, being unable to go out overnight, loss of sleep. In view of these difficulties and their discovery of large areas of unmet need, the researchers concluded that an expansion of social services was urgently required (Maeda et al., 1979). Clearly the laudable level of the national effort to build home help services, which has been made in Japan since the 1960s, still leaves gaps to be filled.

Mix of Closed, Open, and Unorganized Care

The Japanese mix of the three kinds of care deserves closer examination. Just as the Japanese have copied other countries, others may wish to imitate Japan. The rate of institutionalization in Japan remains low, still below 1.5 percent, by comparison with 4.5 percent in the United States. There are three major types of institutions: nursing homes (or homes for the aged), special nursing homes, and moderately priced homes. The number of institutions of all types has increased since October 1972, along with the number of persons admitted (Table 6–6). There is a felt need for

Types of Institutions	Number of Institutions			Number of Persons Admitted		
	1972	1973	1977	1972	1973	1977
Nursing Home	870	890	938	64,148	67,770	71,352
Special Nursing Home	272	350	714	20,368	26,503	55,482
Moderately Priced Home	66	82	143	3,969	5,352	8,954

Source: Adapted from Social Welfare Services in Japan, 1973, 1974 & 1979.

TABLE 6–6. Closed Care in Japan: 1972, 1973, and 1974

more special nursing homes (the functional equivalent of the Hong Kong "care and attention" home), and a five-year plan for additional construction.

In addition to the institutions in Table 6–6, which include some 25 homes for the aged blind, there are private homes for the aged required by law to accommodate more than 10 old persons on a regular basis. In 1976 these private homes for the aged were 73 in number, accommodating 3,928 (Japan Institute, 1978, p. 133).

The quality of care in the homes varies. There are a few model institutions incorporating three levels of care under one roof, such as the Tokyo Metropolitan Institute of Gerontology (TMIG). As a rule, moderately priced homes are superior to the run-of-the-mill public homes, which share some of the negative features of similar institutions in other countries.

The shortage of nurses in Japan means that even the TMIG has not been able to keep all of its geriatric wards open. For some old persons, the proprietary home help industry performs a useful service by providing care in the hospital as well as in the home; however, the fees for such service are too high for the average family, unless covered by third-party payers.

Kyoto

In the Japanese city of Kyoto one of the oldest home care projects known is found in the central district where a cottage silk-weaving industry still holds sway. Under the medical supervision of Horikawa Hospital, incapacitated old persons are nursed at home by family members with the back up of a resident physician and a district nurse who make frequent home visits. This kind of medical back up makes it possible to maintain severely disabled persons in open care, including the incontinent, comatose and mentally ill. Here the Japanese have demonstrated, and over a longer time period than most, that it is possible to maintain any case in open care if the necessary costs are accepted by the family and others.

Day Care and Other Modalities

In addition, the Japanese are experimenting with short-stay hospitalization by admitting bedridden old people to the hospital for up to seven days; this again is copied from Britain and other European countries. There is also a beginning interest in day care (or day hospitalization), once more copying Britain. A small experimental survey of day-care needs, reported at the Tokyo Congress, estimated that seven percent of Japanese aged 65 plus require day care, and an additional 0.5 percent short-stay hospitalization of one week or more. According to the survey report, 14.7 percent of the hospitals replying and 43.6 percent of the nursing homes said they had some day-care services, ranging from one to six days per week. Major barriers to the further expansion of such services are the usual: lack of trained personnel, lack of money, and the necessity to provide transportation. Because of these barriers, the researchers recommend that resources be put into a different modality, that of home health care (Maeda and Kagawa, 1978).

In summary, Japan faces the same problems experienced elsewhere in trying to achieve a proper mix of the three kinds of care. Present institutional facilities, in particular special nursing homes, are insufficient. Considerable concern is felt for the large numbers of bedridden, variously estimated at 350,000 to 400,000 (or 4 percent of the population at risk); a few live alone, and the majority are cared for at home by aging females. Although there is a special financial allowance for families caring for bedfast persons, the amount is small, a kind of token payment. As one Japanese woman in Kyoto explained to me, "I do it out of love for my husband, not the money."

Open Care

Other than model institutions offering three levels of care, the Japanese have shown little interest in developing intermediate housing with built-in services of the kind found in Sweden and elsewhere. This is due in part to the shortage of housing and of land for new housing, as well as the continuing high rate of intergenerational co-residence, the culturally favored solution. There has been a small amount of interest in including facilities for the aged and disabled in new town planning, but the major thrust has been to develop home help services as the principal program for keeping old people in their own or relatives' homes.

We have already traced the growth of home help services from small beginnings and presented data on gaps and unmet needs. We will therefore focus here on additional, supplementary and innovative services which add to the open care system.

Meals on Wheels and Additional Services

There is increasing interest in Meals on Wheels as the next service to be developed after home help. Under the traditional home help pattern, the helper's duties include shopping for food and meals preparation; however, when visits are made only twice weekly for two hours each, this leaves little time for other duties. At present, Meals on Wheels services are still considered to be in an experimental stage, with fewer than 100 facilities involved (Japan Institute, 1978, p. 131).

Additional services include: (1) provision of beds and special equipment; (2) telephone installation and reassurance; (3) temporary personal care; (4) family foster care. Special beds and equipment are generally provided for low-income persons aged 65 and over. Including those supplied on a rental basis, there are reportedly beds and replacement mattresses for about 15,000 persons, with bath tubs and water heaters for about 24,000 (Japan Institute, 1978, p. 130).

Free welfare telephones are a relatively recent service in Japan; by the end of fiscal 1979 plans called for the installation of some 46,000 units. Telephone reassurance services employing older volunteers and neighbors have been developed in urban senior centers.

Temporary personal care services are designed to meet the shortage of home nurses by providing a caretaker or senior companion who is a neighborhood volunteer designated by the municipality. This fits with the continuing Japanese practice of using *Minsei-iin*, volunteers available to help with family problems, under social work direction.

The family foster care program has been in existence since the early 1970s but remains on a very small scale with a total of about 125 persons involved (*Social Welfare Service in Japan*, 1979, pp. 12–17).

Innovative Services

In addition to the services already mentioned, the Japanese have been ingenious in developing a variety of grants and subsidies aimed at shoring up open care. We have already noted that welfare centers for the aged are officially encouraged and construction subsidies granted to local communities or voluntary agencies. As of October 1977, a total of 729 such centers were reported throughout the country. As a rule, personal services are not subsidized, although some consultation is available.

More Japanese older people work than in other countries. It is common for persons who retire from their principal employment to reenter the labor force, often working for a smaller company or in some cases a family business. Japan is wrestling with the problem of upping the retirement age and still leaving slots for younger workers. Meanwhile there are experimental programs both in Tokyo and in rural areas to assist older persons who wish to do other kinds of work after retirement, such as handicrafts.

A related service, in addition to the usual public employment offices, is a special free employment exchange service for the aged, provided by Social Welfare Councils in some prefectures and big cities. In fiscal year 1978, the number of offices of this kind was reported to be 132 (*Social Welfare Services in Japan*, 1979, p. 15). Old people's clubs, special days, and sports programs also receive financial help, usually from local governments.

Less well-known are loans for the cost of repair or additions to houses, tax reduction for those who care for the aged, and the like. Thus, if a family adds a room to its house to accommodate aged parents, it is eligible for financial help. A few local governments have shown an interest in constructing "a pair of houses," or flats, so that families can live with or next door to their aged parents (Maeda, 1975).

Unorganized Care

The Japanese practice of co-residence has meant that, until quite recently, about three-fourths of old people have lived with their adult children. The proportion is lower in Tokyo (68%) and is reportedly declining there and in other large cities. One question is whether the rate of decline is being slowed, and might be slowed further, by the kinds of subsidies and innovative steps we have just discussed. In any case, the proportion in coresidence remains far higher than that reported for the three industrial societies of Denmark, United States, and Britain (Japan Institute, 1978, pp. 118–119; Palmore, 1975, pp. 38–39).

In the past, intergenerational exchanges of affection, wisdom and social services have been carried out within the family system; for those employed by Japanese industries, the employing company has also played a familial, nurturing kind of role. Unfortunately, we have little hard data on the nature of these exchanges within families and parent companies, and the ways in which they may now be changing.

In earlier times the old also performed useful functions in the home, such as housework, care of grandchildren, help with the family business and gardening. Data reported by Palmore (1975) indicate that two-thirds of older Japanese are consulted by their children on family problems, as high as 80 percent when the older person is employed. Will this type of exchange also continue at so high a level?

It is difficult to forecast the future pattern of intergenerational exchanges in Japan. New data are needed to document the specifics of the change process.

Summing Up

Kazuo Aoi, a leading Japanese scholar, in a paper given at the Tokyo Congress (1978), enumerated what he saw as the seven major problems concerning old people in Japan:

1. The subjective health rate decreases as people age, in particular that of aging females;

2. The labor force participation rate of the elderly is higher for Japan than for other developed countries, due in part to low pensions;

3. The co-residence rate in Japan is considerably higher than elsewhere, albeit now declining;

4. The proportion of old people and of old couples who live alone is increasing rapidly;

5. There are sizable numbers of bedridden people, most of them cared for at home by aging females;

6. The suicide rate of Japanese aged is high, especially among aged females;

7. To maintain the ideal Japanese lifestyle—living in the same community among relatives and friends, and working as long as possible—requires more in the way of services and social supports than is presently provided.

The ways in which these problems are approached are of crucial importance in setting goals and future directions. An American political scientist, John Campbell, reported in 1978 how the Japanese government moved over a period of ten or fifteen years from virtually no policy to offering an extensive (and expensive) array of programs for old people. He concludes, however, that the "old people boom" is over in Japan. While expenditures continue to rise, the growth is due mainly to "automatic" factors rather than to new policy initiatives.

Japanese programs for old people, earlier a deficit area, have moved rapidly to a much higher plateau. The question is whether the increasing numbers of older Japanese will push Japan to a plateau that is still higher.

7

Sweden: An Example
of Level 4

Sweden has long been admired by outside observers as an advanced welfare state. The Swedish approach to problem-solving in a highly developed affluent industrial society with an articulated social philosophy has produced a long-term care model for the aging and disabled which has been widely imitated. Hence Sweden has been chosen as an example of Level 4: extension of public services to all parts of the country.

It is not one service alone which has been admired, although the development of an increasingly comprehensive home help modality is clearly a leading attribute to the Swedish system. It is rather the combination of basic health care, housing provision and allowances and a three-tiered retirement system which, along with open care services and options, provides both the necessary tripartite foundation and a range of services found in few other societies.

The overall approach may be characterized as "social engineering"; rational, systematic, and bureaucratic (McRae, 1979). The possibility of injustice to an individual or group, violation of rights, or withholding of entitlements is mitigated by an effective method of intervention, i.e., reliance on the ombudsman, as well as by other control devices (Rosenthal, 1967).

There are parallels to the approach of Britain and other Western European countries, as well as similarities with neighboring Scandinavian countries. Norway in particular has emulated Sweden and, according to one indicator (the number of home help working hours per 1,000 population), may even be exceeding Sweden in the present level of effort. Even though the Swedish effort may have peaked (in the view of some Swedish experts) it still remains the most developed system.

It is essentially a public welfare model, with responsibility for services placed at the local community level. The basic service modality, home help, is available in all 278 communes and receives a 36 percent open-ended subsidy from the central government (Bozzetti et al., 1977; Kahn and Kamerman, 1975, 1977).

A lesser known characteristic of the Swedish approach is the division of responsibility for health and social services between different levels of government, with responsibility for the care of the chronically ill lodged since 1951 at the county council level. In 1963 the county councils took over the previous system of district medical officers and in 1967 assumed responsibility for mental health care. Thus the counties gained authority over most of Swedish medical care (Kane and Kane, 1976; Sidel and Sidel, 1978, 1979).

My personal evaluation, as reported earlier, is that this division of responsibilities between local and county governments tends to result in the same kinds of coordination problems found elsewhere (Little, 1978). However, I also find that assigning long-term medical care to one subsystem facilitated the basic policy decision in the social welfare sector to build no more old age homes. Instead, a striking innovation, in the form of "service houses" or "residential hotels" (a kind of intermediate housing) has been developed as an option for housing the marginal elderly in open care.

Population Projections

Sweden is roughly the size of the state of California. The present population is some 8.2 million people, of whom about 15 percent are 65 and over. The birth rate is expected to continue to fall and longevity to increase. Thus the problem is the one highlighted in United Nations reports: increasing numbers and proportion of the old, and in particular the old-old, the proportion of whom is already 19 percent of old-age pensioners (Table 7–1).

Year	Percentage of Total Population	Total Number of People	Percentage of Old-Age Pensioners Over 80	Total Number Old-Age Pensioners Over 80
1975	15.1	1,249,900	18.1	224,500
1980	16.0	1,352,800	19.3	261,200
1985	16.6	1,423,100	21.1	300,500
1990	16.8	1,460,000	23.3	339,800

Source: Swedish Institute, Old-age care in Sweden, p. 1.

TABLE 7–1. Proportion of Swedish Old-Age Pensioners Aged 65 and Over, 1975–1990

Health/Medical Care

More people surviving to older ages will mean additional pressures on an already expensive medical care sector. Since 1955 all inhabitants of Sweden, including aliens, are covered by a comprehensive national health insurance scheme. The cost of medical care has roughly doubled every five years and now consumes more than eight percent of the Gross National Product. At present the country is divided into seven medical care regions, each of which includes up to six counties which are in turn divided into local health districts, staffed by medical officers and district nurses. Health services are provided at each of the three levels (the region, the county, and the district) (Sidel and Sidel, 1979).

Long-term care is recognized as a medical specialty, a subspecialty of internal medicine, about 75 percent of which has to do with geriatric patients. Overall, the present system is found by the Sidels to be pluralistic, expensive, decentralized, regionalized and under stress (1979).

Housing

There are several housing options available to the Swedish pensioner. Means-tested municipal housing allowances are available. As outlined by McRae (1979), the range of choice includes living in: (1) one's own home; (2) a pensioner's flat; (3) an old-fashioned old-age home, either inadequate or modernized; (4) a "residential hotel" or "service house" or "pensioners' service center"; (5) a cluster complex containing more than one housing type. For those needing medical care there are 40,000 long-term care beds (out of a total 150,000 hospital beds), some in large central nursing home facilities, but most in small peripheral units located in individual communities (Bozzetti et al., 1977).

Income Maintenance

In 1913 Sweden was the first country to introduce a universal old age pension. This has been improved over the years, and in 1946 reached a level high enough for the majority to live on (Bengtsson, 1978). In addition to the basic pension, there has been, since 1959, a supplementary pension (ATP), based on one's income from gainful work. Both are index-regulated with the cost of living.

A third tier of the pension system, added in July, 1976, lowered the retirement age from 67 to 65, and also provided for flexibility in the age of retirement and for partial pensions between 60 and 65. Approximately one-fifth of the population are now pensioners. Sweden is one of the few places where one can move in and out of retirement at will (Thunberg, 1977).

In addition to the basic pension there are other allowances and supplements. Municipal housing allowances have already been mentioned. Fees for health and medical services are uniform and low, with reimbursements for related travel and medications. Transportation services are also subsidized and reimbursed, including payment for taxi services for the old and disabled to get to bus stops.

An old person whose income consists only of the basic pension receives many other services free or at nominal cost. Thus real income is considerably higher than stated monetary income, which is supplemented by a number of socially provided, tax-supported services. In fact, with the income tax at present levels, it may actually be advantageous to be at the basic pension level, rather than several notches higher.

Goals

In 1974 the report of a Swedish Commission on Social Welfare set forth a number of general principles under four primary goals: democracy, equality, solidarity, and security. Intermediate goals included information, accessibility, participation, and a reasonable standard of living.

To achieve these goals, seven basic services were listed:

1. Support for the care and development of the child;
2. Support toward maintenance by cash allowance, counseling, and information;
3. Measures such as domestic help, special services for the handicapped, Meals on Wheels, pedicure, hairdressing and telephone services to facilitate independent living by certain groups (the sick, the old, and the handicapped);
4. Measures to support social interaction, activity and community interplay;
5. Transportation services to increase the freedom of action of certain groups (the elderly, the handicapped, etc.);
6. Counseling and information on social questions, and the intermediation of contacts with authorities;
7. A system of duty officers to cover requirements in all sectors.

All services and institutions should have continuity and flexibility and be conveniently situated.

Clearly, the Swedes do not lack desirable goals, subgoals and principles, which are considered of particular importance in dealing with persons "in the danger zone," such as the aged. Additional principles for the proper and humane care of the elderly have been further articulated by official spokespersons. They include: normalization, self-determination, influence and participation and properly managed activities. Good housing, service, care, and social contacts are viewed as especially important (Von Sydow, 1978).

There is a growing emphasis on "activation" or "self-activation," along with "co-determination"—adding life to years, participating, helping to design programs. In summary:

> The basic aim of old age care is to provide elderly people with a secure economic platform, good housing, an opportunity to obtain services and special care, a sense of community with others and meaningful activities. . . . The overall psychological, physical and social welfare needs of a person are assessed and dealt with in a single context [Swedish Institute, 1978].

This means, *inter alia*, an altered and more nuanced view of the old as individuals belonging to a heterogeneous group.

In setting forth these principles the Swedes confess to a past tendency to over-care, especially in the home help or samaritan services. Over-care is now seen as bad, because it increases dependency and leads to a distortion of service (for example, housecleaning at the expense of a "help to self-help" relationship). Goals for individuals are now more specifically defined in terms of the recipient's preserving and enhancing functional levels in daily living. The principle is: each person who is handicapped by age or illness should have a reasonable chance to improve within the limits of her or his capacity (Von Sydow, 1978).

Goals of Closed Care

The goals of closed care are the same, with greater emphasis on medical treatment. For a "high and effective" standard of treatment in long-term care facilities, a leading physician sees four factors as essential: (1) a pleasant, homelike, cheerful environment, with buildings that have adequate storage space for equipment; (2) excellent medical services, utilizing knowledge from general medicine, social medicine, physiotherapy, and rehabilitative medicine—all orchestrated through team activity; (3) a strong rehabilitation program, based on the concept that the patient should manage his or her own personal needs, and should be given intensive functional training to be able to accomplish this; (4) a hospital milieu providing a full range of activities, including reading circles, sports and games adapted to patients' varying capacities, lectures, films, concerts, and theater. These activities are viewed as important in long-term care facilities, not only in stimulating the patient but also in promoting staff morale (Linder in Bozzetti, 1977).

Open Care

The extent to which goals are achieved and principles implemented may be assessed in a preliminary fashion by examining the development and functioning of the open care system in relation to three key issues: access, types of services offered, and delivery of services, urban and rural.

Access

A public welfare model offers the advantage of a single, visible point of entry to the service system, in the form of the local social welfare office. In fact, there are several points of entry, which in Sweden are well publicized (Table 7–2). In addition, the new service houses are themselves providing a further point of entry not only to residents, but also to other pensioners in the nearby community.

In the service houses pensioners and handicapped persons live in self-contained flats or apartments in buildings designed for recreation, therapy and service programs.

Most have a cafeteria or restaurant in which meals can be obtained at low cost. All have resident staff, including a director (the equivalent of the warden in British sheltered housing), and administrative and clerical personnel. Some also have a resident staff of home helpers.

For example, one well-organized service house which I visisted in Linköping has a ratio of one home helper for every ten residents. Two additional helpers are available for emergencies. Medical services are not built in, but are available on call. Built-in security devices include a switchboard which lights up when a resident has failed to flush the toilet for 12 hours; this alerts the staff to possible problems.

The "security blanket" aspect of such housing appears to be successful for staff and residents alike and has resulted in a significant decrease in the number of demands previously made on the night watch section of the social welfare office.

It is interesting that not all residents utilize the services offered. Nevertheless, help is available when they need it. Community residents also take advantage of the services.

An effort is now being made to develop day care or multi-service centers offering a combination of medical, social and recreational possibilities. In this way there are multiple pathways into the service system for

Need	Benefits	Sponsor(s)	Service Agency
Basic Economic Services	National basic pension equalling 95% of the base amount for single people, 155% for a married couple if both are entitled to basic pension (base amount since January 1976 = 9,700 kronor).	Employers & national gov't	Social Ins. Office
	Pension supplement (for an insured person receiving insufficient ATP or no ATP)	Employers & national gov't	Social Ins. Office
	Wife's supplement (subject to a means test)	Employers & national gov't	Social Ins. Office
Supplementary Security	ATP in proportion to previous earnings	Employers	Social Ins. Office
	Special supplementary pension (STP) for workers (LO sector)	Employers	Workers Ins. Co. (AMF)
	Industrial supplementary pension (ITP) for salaried employees (PTK sector)	Employers	Salaried Employees Ins.Co.
Housing	Municipal housing supplement (subject to means test)	Municipal gov't	Social Welfare Off.
	Pensioner housing (home, hotel, or apartment)	Nat'l & municipal gov'ts & pensioner	Social Welfare Office.
	Home adaptation grants and improvement loans	Nat'l & municipal gov'ts	Social Welfare Off.
Care & Services	Social domestic assistance	Nat'l & municipal gov'ts	Social Welfare Off.
	Municipal transportation service for elderly and disabled	Nat'l & municipal gov'ts	Social Welfare Off.
	Aids (prostheses, invalid chairs, hearing aids, and so on)	County Council & Health Ins. Program	Dist. medical officer, dist. nurse or hospital
	Pedicure	Municipal gov't	Social Welfare Off.
	Home nursing grants	County Council	Dist. nurse or dist. med. officer

Initials used in table are as follows: ATP, national supplementary pensions; STP, supplementary pension; LO, Swedish Conference of Trade Unions; AMF, Labour Market Insurance: ITP, Industrial Supplementary Pension; PTK, Federation of Salaried Employees in Industry and Services; SPP, Swedish Staff Pension Society.

Source: Bengtsson, I. Economic Security in Old Age: Swedish Pension Models. Paper prepared for Seminars on Facing an Aging Society, U.S.A. and Canada, October 1978.

TABLE 7–2. Social Benefits Available to Swedish Old-Age Pensioners, 1978

aging Swedes, plus carefully planned publications and announcements. A typical personal account relates:

> On the day I turned 65 I found a leaflet from the local municipality in my letter box with all of the information of the various financial and social benefits which I had become entitled to as an old age pensioner . . . [lists benefits]. The district nurse and a social worker called at my house and enquired about my health and home comfort. . . . Since I am afflicted with arthritis, they arranged for a home helper to come . . . [Salzer, 1978].

The person who wrote the above account lives in a small city of about 37,000 people near Stockholm.

Type of Services Available

The provision of a variety of social services is viewed as essential. Each municipality is directed to include such services in its planning. Services can be directed at individuals or, alternatively, may consist of collective measures. The services organized and managed by the local social services administration are shown in Table 7–3.

Delivery of Services, Urban and Rural

Services vary somewhat in urban and rural areas and variance is observed also between individual municipalities. The core service of home help is the same in every commune. Other services, such as Meals on Wheels, chiropody, hairdressing, bathing, and personal care cluster around this core. Public transportation is available for the non-handicapped, with special arrangements for the disabled.

Services available on an individual basis:

    Homemaker service which includes: home help; laundry service; Meals on Wheels; chiropody; physical exercise; bathing help; friendly visits; cleaning service; snow-clearing; transportation service; telephone services; technical aids (ADL); hairdressing.

Services available collectively:

    chiropody; hairdressing; bathing help; physiotherapy, physical exercise; library; study groups; hobby activities; restaurant; theater; film; music.

Leisure time activities:

    excursions; study groups; dancing; tours; bookmobiles; singing, theater; film; music, etc.

Source: Von Sydow. Home sweet home, p. 8.

TABLE 7–3. Swedish Social Services, 1978

The home help service is the oldest and by far the largest of the services provided. Home help in a city like Stockholm includes six major components: personal care, shopping, cooking, care of clothes, foot care and housekeeping. Additional services available through the home help organizer include referrals to hobby groups and social clubs, referrals to school lunch programs and the provision of technical aids such as hearing aids or eyeglasses. Clients are encouraged to talk to their home helpers about any personal or practical problems so that a good deal of informal counseling takes place, as well as a reduction of social isolation.

Meals on Wheels are available to the homebound. However, the Swedish service places emphasis on the use of other resources, such as encouraging pensioners to eat their noon meal at local schools. Menus are printed in daily papers. In service houses residents are free to eat as they please at the subsidized cafeterias; many take advantage of this by eating a substantial cafeteria meal at noon, then preparing other meals and snacks in their own flats.

The Swedes have also been successful with service buses, as a complement to the basic home help service. These vans, which are equipped with cleaning supplies, plastic laundry baskets, insulated containers for fresh and frozen food, supplies for hairdressing and shaving, bookcases for books and information material—a veritable smorgasbord—cover one or more districts on a regular schedule. In certain cases a bus is also equipped with a hot plate, iron, ironing board, sewing machine, etc. Usually there are two helpers on duty on each bus; interestingly, it has been possible to recruit more male helpers for this kind of assignment.

Stockholm

A person living in Stockholm, for example, is located in one of 17 social welfare districts, each of which has a social service center. These centers include one or more social welfare sections, plus a domestic service section responsible for providing pensioners with help and advice in matters such as housing.

One which I visited was located in a modern shopping mall, next to a subway station and adjacent to a public housing project which included older residents. Home help assistants (young persons whose varying backgrounds are similar to untrained public welfare workers in the United States) each cover one area. They receive and investigate all referrals for home help service for that area and perform case management functions in organizing and monitoring services. Their supervisor is an experienced administrator and home help organizer. Every referral is said to receive prompt attention; the stated goal of the department is to respond to every perceived need and to serve every known case.

Rural Areas

Rural areas have a slightly different pattern of service, but one which still centers around the core of home help. Service buses often have to cover several districts, but may cover only one if the aged population there is scattered and socially isolated.

Essentially the same services are available as in urban areas. However, it is admittedly more difficult to provide the same coverage as in urban areas with clusters of older people.

The Rural Postman

An innovative program is the use of rural postmen to supply certain services to old people in sparsely populated places. In 1974, after some discussion and small-scale testing, the Post Office (which was having budgetary problems) concluded an agreement with the National Board of Health and Welfare. This specified that rural postmen would carry out the following social services: contact and alarm, goods delivery, home visits, plus special duties. In making this agreement the Post Office had several bargaining points: a detailed map of every municipality, showing the location of each dwelling, plus the availability of a person who regularly covered these roads and knew those living on his route.

Municipalities have the option to extend their social services by making a contract with the Post Office Department and paying a fixed monthly fee for agreed services. Some municipalities are not interested in goods delivery, which may already be covered by shopmobiles; hence contracts vary. If more than 12 home visits or special duties are needed in one month, the payment of an additional fee may be specified.

The service is useful because it provides contact and security for elderly and isolated persons. Home visits and special duties (which are usually of a "look in" or "call with the mail" nature) have proved useful for persons who are ill or recently discharged from hospital. The postman meets once monthly with the social worker to report contacts and review situations which may require additional service.

Mix of Closed, Open, and Unorganized Care

The Swedes themselves judge the effectiveness of elderservices largely by the numbers of old persons maintained in open care, in which they include the residents of service houses. However, as in other countries, there is a mix of closed, open, and some unorganized care to be examined.

It is reported that approximately eight percent of Swedes aged 70 and over are in homes for the aged, with four percent in various kinds of nursing homes or long-term care facilities. In total numbers this amounts to some 90,000 persons receiving some type of institutional care (Bozzetti et al., 1977). The great majority of people aged 65 or over (88 percent) live in ordinary dwellings, single family houses or apartments.

In 1977 there were some 30,000 pensioners' flats. In addition, there were about 12,500 apartments in 157 service buildings. The new modality of service housing thus cares for about one percent of people aged 70 plus. Additional service houses are being built and more are planned. However, there are also long waiting lists, reportedly as high as 6,000 in Stockholm (McRae, 1979). Overall, it is estimated that about three percent of older pensioners live either in pensioners' flats or service houses (Von Sydow, 1978).

In Sweden home help has been used not only as a service but as a collective concept for different kinds of activity. In 1977 about 70,000 home helpers provided services to some 300,000 elderly people. A survey reported that nine percent of pensioners between 65 and 74 received home help; 26 percent of those between 75 and 80; and 40 percent of those aged 80 and over. As the population at risk ages, the numbers and proportion of recipients increase.

This same survey reported that 11 percent of the recipients would like more help. Some 14 percent would prefer to move, usually to an apartment, but less than half have done anything about it. About two percent reportedly want to move to service housing, and one percent want to move to homes for the aged. It seems that there are still some gaps, deficits, and problems in the most highly developed and diversified open care system we have studied.

Labor Pool

Traditional home help, in Sweden and elsewhere, has relied on a largely untrained labor force, typically middle-aged housewives. This marginal labor pool may be drying up just at the time that the frail elderly population at risk is increasing. How to recruit, train, and expand the labor force is thus seen as a major emerging problem.

Here Sweden is considering following the example of Netherlands, West Germany, and other Western European countries by defining home help as a "profession" and then training secondary school graduates, both male and female, in a one- to two-year course which combines practical and classroom instruction. This kind of planned labor pool expansion would be more costly in resource terms and would require both larger budgetary allocations for training programs and higher rates of pay for more skilled and experienced workers. A career ladder would have to be provided as a further incentive. In less obvious ways, it might reduce the serendipitous gains from what Bozzetti et al. (1977) term the "functional" or "contractual" reciprocity of the present system; by this they mean utilizing the maternal ethic of the helpers, who serve as loving daughter figures to parental surrogates, with psychological gains for both in the relationship.

Home Help as the Core Service

Home help continues to be the core service around which other services cluster. Assigning a staff of home helpers to a service house is one method of making an individual service collective, and is proving more cost-efficient, like the service buses.

The Swedes are also experimenting with decentralization and various kinds of team arrangements, some with medical as well as social components, and different patterns of leadership. For example, a team of 15 to 20 is responsible for some 50 pensioners; they work out of a central office, where they meet daily to plan their activities, often working in pairs. These experiments are still in the early stages.

Unorganized Care

Little is known of unorganized care in Sweden. The general belief is that it doesn't exist. A three-generation family is considered a rarity. According to most accounts, the industrialization of Sweden meant the movement of the young and economically active to urban areas, leaving older people behind in rural areas, often without family supports. American studies by Shanas and others have found that a majority of older Americans live within an hour's distance of one of their adult children, and that interpersonal contacts are frequent. This kind of information is not available for Sweden. Concern is felt about loneliness and depression, alcoholism and social isolation as problems of older Swedes. There are said to be infrequent family visits, sometimes only once a year at Christmas time. Here again more data are needed.

A basic issue is whether social provision in fact reduces family care. The Swedes say, "We pay strangers to take care of old people; why not pay their families, who would give them better care?" It is reported that, in addition to the 70,000 home helpers, 20,000 family members are also being paid for care of the old. This does not indicate whether other families in fact rely on publicly provided services, but is in line with the approach of Britain, Japan and other developed countries which provide family respite or back-up services such as housing subsidies, income tax relief, special equipment, laundry service, short-stay hospitalizations, family vacations, and the like.

Human and Cost Effectiveness

The Swedes are convinced that their care system is both human and cost effective, and they feel that it could be made even more humanly effective in enhancing the quality of life for pensioners. Goals such as self-activation and co-determination cannot be achieved overnight.

I pointed out earlier (Little, 1978) that data are lacking to measure cost-effectivenesss in a precise way. What we now have are input data which show a steady increase in numbers of helpers, numbers of cases served, hours of service delivered, diversity of services, new programs, and the like. The Swedes also cite partial cost figures, which suggest that the cost to municipal budgets of maintaining a frail person in a service house is less than it would cost to maintain that same person in a nursing home. According to Bozzetti et al. (1977), it may be only half the cost. As I pointed out earlier, however, following the reasoning of Doherty and Hicks (1975), this fails to include the whole range of primary, secondary, tertiary, and hidden social costs involved.

Swedish leaders themselves admit that they lack data to evaluate the service house modality properly. It is not clear, for example, to what extent different levels of care can and will be provided, as present residents age. In fact, service housing might also be organized in ordinary apartment houses, avoiding the disadvantages of age segregation.

One indicator of the effectiveness of service which I use is: what proportion of the eligible population is reached? Many open care systems reach only one percent to two percent, which is low, considering that the disabled elderly represent 20 percent to 25 percent of the total. According to their own estimates, Swedish services in Stockholm reach one out of every three pensioners which, if accurate, is high. Some of the services are recreational, cultural and educational and are aimed at a much larger target group of potential participants.

A second indicator is: what proportion of the population at risk are at the appropriate level of care? In many countries, severely incapacitated and bedfast elderly are found in unorganized care in the community, whereas fairly active, mobile, and only slightly incapacitated persons are found in closed care. Theoretically, the availability of open care in Sweden, coupled with the availability of long-term care beds, should result in a more rational allocation of aging individuals to the appropriate level of care. Again, data are lacking.

Sweden as a Model?

Sweden may well be an imperfect model, but it is the best example we have of a rational, public provision approach. It may not be the choice of other industrial societies which are more polyglot, less rational, more averse to taxes, and which lack the Swedish philosophy that a civilized society is measured by the quality of life made possible for all of its members.

Professional concerns have tended to focus on the areas of the mental health status and life satisfaction of aging Sweden. In most societies there appears to be a bad marriage between industrialization and aging. Man-in-the-street criticisms, on the other hand, tend to focus on the level of taxation. One estimate is that the average taxpayer in Stockholm pays the following income taxes: national, 25 percent, county council, 13 percent, and municipal, 11 percent. In addition, there is a "marginal tax," which could amount to 75 percent of the last SKr 3,000 one earns, depending on total annual income (Bozzetti et al., 1977). Many retired persons, however, are entirely exempt from taxes. A pensioner is not assessed for taxes if his/her income does not exceed a normal old age pension plus SKr 3,800 a year, including pension supplements. Municipal housing allowances, other housing subsidies and disability allowances are not taxed.

All old age pensions and services represent a kind of intergenerational transfer, based on an assumed reciprocity so that when the present young become old they, too, will receive from their descendants. However, it is difficult to calculate in numerical terms what the present transfer amounts to and even more difficult to predict the future. If the quality of life is valued, and the European standard of equity between the generations maintained, the resource cost of the transfer is bound to increase.

Thoughtful students have raised other questions equally difficult to answer. McRae, for example, finds praiseworthy the strong social consciousness in the Scandinavian countries he has studied, such as Sweden, and feels that their housing programs are beginning to achieve the goal of continued independence for pensioners. Overall he finds a broad, well-meaning and, in most cases, excellent approach. However, this approach conceals a number of problems, such as: when does "self care" become welfare? How does the "social supermarket" achieve flexibility and sensitivity to changing needs? How can a society avoid a "get-an-idea-and-stamp-it-out" approach with older people (McRae, 1979)?

My own final question is: Is this indeed the way we would choose to live as old people in an affluent society?

Part III

Issues and Problems in Open Care

8

The Family as a Unit of Care

Having examined the care mix in four societies at different levels of open care development, we now turn our attention to the major issues and problems which all systems face, beginning with the family as a unit of care.

In all societies there are human networks of persons related by blood, marriage, love, friendship, propinquity and other ties. All of the world's major religions prescribe caring for one's neighbor. Hence mutual aid is normal.

Mutual aid between old people and their adult children is also a universal norm. It does not cease to operate as economies become more technologized, even though it may be less visible. In Western countries there has been a secular tendency for families to yield to bureaucracies functions which can be made uniform and routinized, such as health, education, and welfare. In the case of eldercare, however, a sharing of functions is more usual. In fact, the family participates in open and closed, as well as unorganized, care, and is in every country the basic unit of care, performing linkage, mediating and coordinating functions as well as supplying both expressive and instrumental services (Shanas and Streib, 1965; Shanas and Sussman, 1977).

Who does what for whom? What are the behavioral and legal norms? What is the incentive structure? These questions are largely unanswered. Historically, public social welfare came into being because of gaps in family systems. Both historically and currently, frail elderly lacking family supports tend to be placed in closed care.

Is greater community provision to supplement the inadequacies of family care the hallmark of an advanced stage of development? The answer used to be "Yes," but present thinking is that perhaps family back-up or respite services, as well as finding and organizing natural networks, may be the first line of defense. A limited amount of evidence suggests that family care may drop off when social agencies take over; at the same time, agencies fold their tents and silently steal away when families seem to be coping. Hence the distinction between familial and societal responsibility remains blurred and indistinct. According to Weihl, the problem is more fundamental: without an accepted value position neither family nor society will allocate resources to the old (Weihl in Shanas and Sussman, 1977).

As we have already noted, myths and stereotypes prevail; some of them are propagated by academics. For example, there is the prevailing belief that the multigenerational family of the past contracted to become the nuclear family of today. This belief was nourished by generations of sociologists but is now questioned by modern research, which finds that the three-generation family as a unit of co-residence never really existed at a substantially higher rate than it does today, at least in Western countries (Laslett, 1972). A second myth is that Oriental societies love and revere the old, whereas youth-oriented cultures, such as the United States, discard them like used tin cans. The latter myth has its scholarly proponents, and is just beginning to be tested by data.

Some are now engaged in creating a new myth, the myth of natural networks. Surveys find that the majority of old persons in any country are linked with their kin and with caring others. However, we also know that there are subgroups at special risk, such as: (1) singletons, without living relatives or significant others; (2) old-old, who have outlived their relatives; (3) those separated from relatives by geography and political events; (4) those with relatives who care poorly, or not at all; (5) those with divisive family conflicts, which lead to separation and often to closed care. The historic joint or extended family, serving as its own social security system, may well be less able to cope, as we have already seen in the case of Western Samoa.

Family Care in the United States

Not only in Samoa, but also in the United States, the family remains the basic unit of care providing, according to current estimates, up to 80 percent of the care received by older Americans. The myth that families do not care has been attacked by a number of scholars, led by Shanas (1962, 1968, 1971, 1974). Her original survey, part of the studies of the United States, Denmark and Britain as three industrial societies, had been repeated twice, in 1965 and 1975. Her most recent report reiterates the earlier major findings. About three percent of the 1975 sample of noninstitutionalized elderly were classified as bedfast and seven percent as housebound, a total of 10 percent, twice that of the institutionalized (Shanas, 1979).

Who cares for the bedfast and homebound? The main source of help is the husband or wife of the invalid, with some assistance by paid helpers. Children within and outside of the household are the next main source of help. Two-thirds of the men who reported being ill in bed one day or more were taken care of by wives; women, more likely to be widowed, were taken care of by children in one-third of the cases. However, one of every four persons who reported being ill in bed one or more days had no help at all, especially if that person was a woman (Shanas, 1979, Tables 3 and 4).

Further evidence of the family role in caring for very impaired old people is found in an official report to the Congress by the Comptroller-General of the United States (1977). Using a Cleveland, Ohio, sample, the researchers found that 14 percent of the elderly living at home were greatly or extremely impaired, and were getting care at home the equivalent of that in institutions. They concluded that at all impairment levels family and friends provide 50 percent of the services received by old people and over 70 percent of the services received by the impaired.

What about the silent majority of old people who are not significantly impaired? Here the attention of Shanas and other researchers has focused on evidence of interaction, such as the visiting patterns of old people and their adult children. For 1975 Shanas reports more than half of old persons with surviving children had seen one of their children either the day they were interviewed or on the day before that. Three of every four persons with children saw one of their children within the week's period preceding the interview; about one person in 10 had last seen one more than a month before the interview.

When children were not seen during the previous week, about four of every 10 saw a brother or sister or other relative. About 13 of every 100 old people have no surviving children. For these persons there is some evidence that brothers, sisters and other relatives tend to substitute for a child (Shanas, 1979, Tables 5 and 6).

Additional data are available from the Harris survey commissioned by the National Council on the Aging (1975). The overall results are similar to those reported by Shanas. However, as analyzed by Mahoney (1977), there are significant community differences in five major areas: existence of children, shared residence with children, frequency of face-to-face contact with children, assistance and advice from children, and existence of close relationships. For example, suburban elderly are the most likely to have children, to move in with their children and to interact with them most frequently. Rural elderly are more likely to have five or more children and to receive the greatest total of different kinds of advice.

Urban aged, according to Mahoney, appear to be less assisted and more socially isolated. This fits with other findings. A study of personal time dependency (PTD) in New York City defined the concept as "the state of dependency requiring time-consuming help from another person." The researchers found that the PTD elderly and their families were predisposed to depression, with depression warranting clinical attention occurring in at least one in eight cases of elderly persons with PTD, and one in four households in which a PTD person resides. For this highly dependent group, formal support personnel (nurses, aides, home helpers) provided about 15 percent of primary support services and daughters, spouses, and other family members about 77 percent. There was little assistance from friends.

Further evidence of the role of the family and informal support in caring for a low-income inner-city New York sample is reported by Cantor and Johnson (1978). Two-thirds had immediate kin defined as "functional," either because they were co-resident or because they were in regular contact. Another 18 percent had kin, either a sibling or other relative. Only 15 percent were without at least one functional kin and these were more apt to receive both affective and instrumental support from friends and relatives. Only 14 percent of the entire sample lacked visible informal supports.

Family Care in Other Countries

Cross-national comparisons of residential proximity find that 88 percent of old people in Poland, 82 percent in Great Britain, and 75 percent in Denmark have children living no more than half an hour away in travel time, compared with 77 percent in the United States. By contrast, for about a quarter or a fifth of the elderly in the Netherlands, the geographic distance between parents and children is so large that the child cannot help in case of emergency (Munnichs in Shanas and Sussman, 1977).

In France the proportion of elderly people with no children living in the neighborhood varies from 29 percent for farmers to 41 percent for city dwellers to 68 percent for non-farm rural. Paradoxically, as Paillat points out, parental fertility is such a strong factor in migration that a couple with many children may find themselves even more isolated in old age than couples with fewer children (Paillat in Shanas and Sussman, 1977).

As a rule, older people prefer not to live with children, but poor health, low income, or widowhood may lead them to do so. In poor countries with housing shortages, often combined with inadequate or no pensions, the old may have no other option. In the United States the number of separate households headed by an older person has increased significantly since the passage of the Social Security Act in 1935; however, according to Carp, the growing tendency of the old to prefer, and to occupy, separate households can be traced as far back as the Middle Ages (Carp in Binstock and Shanas, 1976).

For the Netherlands, Munnichs further reported a large increase between 1960 and 1970 in the total elderly living independently, both as heads of households and as single persons living alone, along with decreases in those sharing their household with others, or living in other people's households. A sizable number preferred (after remaining in their own homes) in case of emergency to move to an old age home or to social housing; only 1.7 percent wanted to move in with their own children. A similarly low percentage answered "Yes" to the question, "Would you like to live with one of your married children?" (Munnichs in Shanas and Sussman, 1977).

Intimacy at a Distance

More empirical data are found in the Austrian studies of Leopold Rosenmayr and associates, one a 1971 microcensus and the second a 1972 public opinion sampling. These data support his earlier finding that the general tendency toward separate households is not an irrevocable detachment, but rather a preference for "intimacy at a distance." The wish to live closer to the children is, however, negatively correlated with the size of the community.

As Rosenmayr sees it, joint living is caused primarily by economic needs. In smaller communities, especially those with fewer than 2,000 inhabitants, older religious traditions persist and tend to exert continuing pressure for joint living. Over time, modern intergenerational structures tend toward an optimal mix of intimacy and distance. Extreme closeness and extreme distance do not attract more than relatively small minorities (Rosenmayr in Shanas and Sussman, 1977).

Types of Help

The Austrian researchers have also collected data on three categories of intergenerational help patterns: (1) help in the household, (2) assistance with shopping, and (3) nursing in case of sickness. They find that women tend to receive more help than men, and persons living alone significantly more help than those living with others. However, only one of five persons 60 and over living alone receives any household help at all. For the sample as a whole more than 90 percent of males and almost the same proportion of females receive help less than once a week or never.

Help with daily shopping is almost twice as frequent as help with housekeeping, again going most often to aged women living alone in small

communities. A similar pattern is found for expectations of nursing help
when ill. Rosenmayr concluded that the degree of help desired by the
elderly equalled the amount the younger generation was willing to give
and actually gave. As with formal open care services, the supply establishes
the demand, rather than vice versa.

Limits to Natural Networks

There are limits to the amount and kind of help which families give their
aging parents. Even more limited help is given by nonrelatives. The
perception of these limits both increases the willingness of the old to enter
closed care and at the same time exerts pressure on governments to
increase open care and family back-up services.

Not a great deal is known about family care, and even less about other
informal support systems. The network of a specific older person may be
strong, tenuous, or nonexistent. Just as formal institutions and agencies
vary in the quality of care offered, so do families, neighbors and friends. A
data base is just beginning to emerge, and Silverstone reports a variety of
early findings, some fragmentary, others conflicting (Silverstone, 1978).

Silverstone concludes that informal supports are important but
seriously questions whether they can fill the service gap. For a variety of
reasons individual families reach a point of no return in coping with an
aging parent at home, and institutionalization usually follows. "Perceived
inconvenience" is the most predictive factor. In view of the high prevalence of depression in dependent elders and their households, it seems
that many families continue over long periods of time, at heavy psychic
cost, in situations which the economist Kenneth Boulding once termed
"sacrifice traps."

Lurie agrees with Silverstone that there are indeed limits, but that we
know too little about informal supports as yet to specify them in more than a
preliminary way. She lists inconsistency of values, role strain, and mental
health of supporters as constraints, in addition to financial and activity
constraints. Both formal and informal systems experience strain in meeting
the continuous needs of frail old persons. For the immediate future, formal
systems are seen as complements to informal. However, the questions
which need empirical answers are: *why, who, how well,* and *how better*
(Lurie, 1979).

9

Assessing the Needs
of the Elderly

If the family is the unit of care, it is also the unit of needs assessment. When an older person enters the formal structure of open care, assessment is done by the provider. Whatever the approach, there is danger that the older person's own perceptions of need will be distorted and devaluated.

Hence, assessing the needs of the elderly is an art with many facets. The state of the art is presently in its infancy. Need is a multidimensional concept. What is a need? Who decides?

Needs perceptions, like beauty, vary with the eye of the beholder; they are relative to person, time, place, culture, and rising expectations.

There is an apparent tension between a humanist, people-oriented approach, starting from the belief that there are "common human needs," and a political economy approach which assumes that, because of resource scarcity and fiscal constraints, only a portion of known needs will be met from public funds (Little, 1980–1981).

The needs of the elderly may be classified in various ways. Berkman and Rehr (1972) defined and categorized the social needs of the hospitalized elderly, using reasons for referral to social service. A carefully worked out classification of nine discrete need areas, each with five scaled levels measuring from one (little need, independent) to five (high need, dependent) was part of the design of a comprehensive study of aging in Manitoba. This represented the collapse of an initial eighteen areas, identified from the literature, previous surveys and studies, professional opinions, and selective feedback from elderly persons (Province of Manitoba, 1973).

Varying Perceptions of Needs

Without defining or categorizing needs many surveys proceed on a "within the system" basis, listing various services (either existing or known) and asking old persons which they feel a need for. When these same questions are asked of others, significant differences are found in the responses given.

A Danish gerontologist, Ole Svane, investigating elderly people's need for nursing and care in five neighboring municipalities, found wide variations (from 5 percent to 25 percent) in the amount of home help supplied to persons aged 70 and over. Even more interesting, he found that the aged person's own assessment of his/her unmet need for home help differed from the interviewer's assessment, which differed from the social authorities' assessment. The G.P.'s and the aged person's own assessments were typically low whereas the interviewer's were highest, followed by the social authorities'. When the four unmet needs assessments are averaged for each of the five municipalities, the result if surprisingly stable, about eight percent.

After analyzing possible explanations for the variance, Svane concluded that the most decisive seemed to be "the proportion of home help granted at the time of the investigation." Once more, supply establishes demand.

Similar differences among the four assessing groups were found in their estimates of unmet need for institutional accommodation for persons aged 70 and over. Svane concluded:

> The most important result of this analysis is that the supply of welfare services offered by a given municipality seems to be of vital importance in assessing the total need. It is supposed that an increase in the supply will entail that new groups of elderly people will be considered to be in need of help [Svane, 1973].

Further evidence on varying needs perceptions has been developed by Eva Kahana and associates in studies of two ethnic neighborhoods in the Detroit area. Comparing "significant others" with older persons' and service agencies' perceptions, Kahana found differences of both degree and kind. Older people perceived greater service needs among the aged than did significant others. Expressions of personal need among the aged were also higher than that attributed to significant others. Among service needs voiced by the aged, housing was the number one priority. The agencies and significant others perceived greater need for emotional support or psychological help than was acknowledged by respondents themselves. There was overall consensus, however, on the primary importance of financial assistance and health services.

Kahana went on to analyze the intercorrelations among various needs, as well as the dimensionality of service needs. Expressed needs for domestic maintenance (laundry, repairs, cooking) were found to be intercorrelated with other needs, such as health, self-maintenance and financial problems, whereas personal care difficulties appeared to be independent of all others, except for domestic maintenance. Even for relatively healthy older persons living in the community, Kahana concluded that there was a great deal of overlap in areas of need, unmatched by available services which tend to be isolated "Band-aid" offerings (Kahana, 1974; Kahana and Fairchild, 1976).

Similar issues have been addressed by Gottesman, Moss, and other researchers at the Philadelphia Geriatric Center in the so-called Logan Project. In a 1975 paper they reported considerable congruence in the responses of the older person about himself and that of his significant relative with regard to actual functioning, with more discrepant judgments about potential functioning. There was more disagreement and uncommon agreement in their respective opinions as to which of 20 listed services might be needed. The research team concluded that there was no pattern of congruence, but rather a *persistence* of incongruence. Like others, they found that older persons needed more health and instrumental assistance, while relatives saw the need for more psychosocial services (Moss et al., 1975a).

In a later paper (1975b) they presented additional data on questionnaire-elicited needs and wants as perceived by respondents, compared with clinical judgments by a nurse-social worker team, and the estimates of outreach workers. Here the researchers found that the questionnaire elicited more than half of the wants in each category. Clinical review generally added medical care services and social supports. The outreach staff was particularly perceptive of additional needs for concrete functional services, such as Meals on Wheels, housework, and transportation.

A further significant finding is that needs and wants change over time. When queried several months later, old persons said that they did not want 27 percent of the services they initially desired. With regard to utilization, about three-fourths were receptive to outreach service, one-third of whom were judged as "high need" and two-thirds as "low need."

Monk and Cryns (1976) have also been interested in the relationship between varying perceptions of service needs and intended utilization of services. They found in a blue collar Buffalo neighborhood that desire for services was, in most instances, higher than the admission of need; the services most wanted were transportation and home repairs. Their profile of the high needer is: an elderly person who has health and mobility problems, tends to be financially dependent, often lacks suitable transportation, and yet is positively cathected to maintaining his lifestyle.

In an earlier study of two groups of rural administrators—service providers and public officials—they found agreement on the major problems (lack of transportation, lack of knowledge about services), but a distinct tendency for providers to see the obstacles to better service as significantly greater, and existing services as less adequate to the expressed demand, than did the administrators (Monk and Cryns, 1975).

Another study found that the perceptions of service providers vary with their amount of training in gerontology, regardless of the age and income levels of those served. In this study administrators' perceptions of needs had greater congruence with those of the elderly than the perceptions of workers in the field (Avant and Dressel, 1976).

Methods of Assessment

Conceptual approaches to assessment may be categorized as *rational, empirical,* or *relativistic.* The *rational* approach is a professional estimate of the deviation from an ideal state of well-being and is more comprehensive, but also more biased. The *empirical* approach measures actual demand at the current utilization level (that is, the status quo), assuming that people below an average level demand automatically and are supplied. The *relativistic* approach is based on a process of consensus-building in the community, and is considered politically realistic, although possibly over-influenced by providers at the expense of consumers.

Whichever approach is chosen, the assessor must still make a series of decisions about how to measure needs. For example, he or she must choose between *objective* measures such as low income and *subjective* (ask the person if he needs the service). The subjective definition of the situation is influenced by social-psychological perceptions as well as by political processes and may, as previously suggested, differ noticeably from that of significant others, professionals and administrators.

Methodologies now employed often combine or mix conceptual and objective-subjective approaches. Because of the pressures on planners, a cookbook-type literature is springing up, which tells how to do it—or how it was actually done in Kansas City (Project SHARE, 1976). There seems to be emerging agreement, however, among researchers in several countries, that no one method will do; the crudeness of much of the data mandates a multifaceted approach.

The Survey Method

The oldest method known, and still the most frequently used in this and other countries, is the social survey—essentially a research technique for selecting and interviewing a sample from within a given universe. The validity of the results varies with the efficacy of the design and the competence of the interviewers.

Peer interviews by trained senior citizens have been used with success in some instances, such as an earlier (1971) study in Vermont. More recently, in Wethersfield, Connecticut, some 20 volunteers were given six hours of training and successfully completed a survey of elderly needs, although the refusal rate was high (Wethersfield, 1977). Interviewing by trained and supervised students is another commonly used method. In March 1978 the Hong Kong Council of Social Service completed its first comprehensive research project, using 30 students from the Chinese University to interview a sample of 808 respondents.

The Search for a Common Instrument

All around the world needs are assessed on different levels (individual, group, state, province, nation, universe), almost always using different instruments. There is an unfortunate tendency for each new project to reinvent the wheel and make up its own interview form; the resulting information is then not comparable with that gathered elsewhere by other methods. However, some progress is being made in refining and sharing instruments. A notable example is the Cross-National Geriatric Community Study in which two teams, one in New York and one in London, are working on a comprehensive assessment and referral evaluation (CARE) which has been tested with more than 850 community residents aged 65 and over in the two countries (Gurland et al., 1977–1978).

A good example of a statewide project is that of Lawrence Branch, who has been refining the instrument he designed in order to build a body of data on the health and social service needs of people aged 65 and over in the State of Massachusetts (Branch, 1977). A provincial project, already noted, is the study of aging in Manitoba; the Manitoba instrument has also been used in Montreal, Cleveland, Finland, Tel Aviv, Prince Edward Island, and Connecticut.

The Older American Status and Needs Assessment Survey used by several American states, including Maine and Vermont, was also employed for the cross-national study with Japan, previously discussed.

Criticisms of the Survey Method

As the Japanese project demonstrated, the survey information is incomplete unless nonrecipients are included as well as recipients. Recipients are apt to be biased in favor of the services they are now utilizing or, in some cases, afraid that if they are critical, the services will be withdrawn or curtailed.

The survey method is criticized on other grounds. It is expensive, and the refusal rate is high, both in the United States and Japan. Some savings can be effected through telephone rather than in-person interviews, but it remains a time-consuming process, with the results often outdated by the time the report is completed. Branch solved this problem by doing a second study at Time 2, updating the Time 1 results and revising his operational definitions. The Manitoba project faced the same problem, and came up with a shorter, less expensive way of updating its findings, using field workers with no special training.

Other Methods

Due to the fiscal and practical problems in conducting extensive field surveys, planners are turning to other methods, sometimes copying those developed in the mental health field, such as the key informant, the Delphi, modified Delphi, or the community forum approach. For example, a well conducted United Way survey in Bridgeport, Connecticut, defined "community needs" as: gaps between the current frequency or severity of a community social problem and the level which people think is appropriate, given existing human services technology. They then distinguished "high," "medium," and "low" need programs, according to the ranking of the various groups surveyed (United Way of Eastern Fairfield County, 1977).

In the absence of epidemiological data about possible target populations, various approximations are employed, such as the use of social indicators. Spurred by the Federal Administration on Aging, 34 states completed Social Indicators needs assessment projects; unfortunately, over half modified or substituted instruments, so there was a loss of comparable nationwide data.

The aggregate or gross countdown method is common in local studies. Here one begins with national data on incidence and prevalence rates, and extrapolates from larger to smaller units. Census data are available and the U.S. Bureau of the Census has, since 1976, conducted studies aimed at augmenting user orientation; in the process, it has developed social statistics for the elderly at the state, area, and city levels, available on request (Wallach, 1977). Now that a national census is to be taken at five- instead of ten-year intervals, it may be possible to improve its adequacy in critical areas (Kendig and Warren, 1976).

On a smaller scale, client analysis (an empirical approach) may be done fairly simply, using current utilization figures and recorded waiting lists. Some local authorities in England have used this method and it has also been employed by city planners in Tokyo.

A variant of the "existing services" approach is to ask a group of people which services they need or would use if available. When this was done in northeastern Connecticut, the consultant found *inter alia* that some 1,300 elderly persons had transportation needs and 4,300 home maintenance needs. The greatest need, however, was for "attention and companionship" (McKain, 1975).

Statistical manipulation, displaying computer capability, dominates the scene. Rather than a laundry list of possible services, a matrix or problem-service taxonomy is developed, or an activity sector/target population framework. An effort is made to operationalize program goals and objectives; sometimes the UWASIS (United Way Services Identification System) is used to delineate service areas.

The most highly developed statistical techniques, both in Britain and the United States, are methods of dealing with SMSAs (Standard Metropolitan Statistical Areas) and relating a group of variables to a known benchmark measure; regressive equations and/or discriminant functions are then employed. This method helps to pinpoint areas of special need within a given catchment area and leads to formulas for the allocation of funds according to relative percentages of need. Its technical impressiveness may rest, however, on little or no subjective data and dubious assumptions about age-related changes. It fails to deal with the known heterogeneity of aging cohorts and the fact of increasing individual differences with age.

An interesting variant, where there is computer capability, is that developed earlier for planning elderly services in Manchester, England. It could be termed a "representative cases" approach. The technique requires a management information system (MIS) which will yield detailed data on client characteristics. From this can be abstracted a certain number of typical situations whose established frequency may be used as a basis for planning services aimed at these kinds of situations (Manchester, England, 1972).

Computer capability may also be employed to establish a service preference model, which will help to distinguish the present and future preferences of aging persons living in different types of communities (Mahoney, 1976). In this way, many service and demonstration projects are launched on a wing and a prayer, based on computer-reinforced educated guesses as to needs and potential utilization patterns. The universal hope is that a new service will catch on and will generate enough data to permit monitoring, feedback, evaluation and revision. This requires the installation of a basic data recording and retrieval system, never an easy task.

Index of Incapacity

A most useful approach to assessing elderly needs is the "index of incapacity" measure, developed by Shanas et al. for their studies of aging in three industrial societies (1968). As noted, these have since been replicated in three other countries (Poland, Israel, and Yugoslavia) and a revised instrument has been used to resurvey the United States. It is a simpler version of ADL (Activities of Daily Living) scales, now widely employed in hospital and clinical work and beginning to be used by community based assessment teams.

This approach is based on the belief that the self-reports of old people as to what they can and cannot do are reliable and yield firm data as to the percent of community dwellers who are bedfast, housebound and/or otherwise in need of services. The respondent is asked a series of simple questions such as: Can you walk? Go up and down stairs? Go outdoors? Bathe, feed, and clothe yourself? Cut your own toenails? If the sample is a good one, the results will give a benchmark measure for home health needs which may then be used as a first step in planning.

This approach has proved adaptable to other cultures and ethnic groups. For example, the study of aging in Manitoba distinguished nine activities in which difficulty might be encountered: doing light housework, doing heavy housework, making a cup of tea or coffee, preparing a hot meal, shoveling and yardwork, shopping, managing financial matters, laundry, and finally, major house or household repairs. Each activity is linked to possible services which might be provided according to need. The sum total of responses provides a data base for planning which is more service-linked than the simpler measures of incapacity. As we have seen in examining the family as a unit of care, these data need supplementation as to who usually helps and who would help in certain contingencies.

The New Zealand Example

An offical New Zealand study on the accommodation and service needs of the elderly illustrates the use of several methodologies, including a variant of the index of incapacity. Essentially a survey, it did a comprehensive job of interviewing and both social and environmental assessment.

Using the individual disability data, the research team constructed a five-point general disability scale, as follows: Class I, Not disabled; Class II, Slightly disabled; Class III, Seriously disabled; Class IV, Mentally disabled; Class V, Severely disabled. In usage it was found more practical to combine Classes III and V.

Service needs were initially assessed at two levels, "essential" and "desirable," but the latter was later dropped as being beyond the scope of potential community resources. Assessed need at the essential level was then calculated on the basis of the ratios of numbers needing the service to 1,000 elderly. The results are seen in Table 9–1. Home aid and day ward care are the areas with the largest deficits, followed by occupational therapy and social day care and laundry service. The only service for which 100 percent of the need is being met is domiciliary nursing.

Although the researchers in New Zealand modestly characterize their estimates as "crude" they have succeeded in producing a set of planning guidelines expressed as ratios per 1,000 elderly and then have gone on to calculate the percentage of known need now being met.

Summing Up

In summary, it may be said that the state of the needs assessment art is in its infancy, with an unclear heritage and fundamental issues of priorities unsettled. While many struggle with different approaches and strive to come up with better methods, most tend to proceed in a far less innovative manner. The New Zealand and Manitoba examples are, unfortunately, few and far between.

Services	Assessed Need Per 1,000 Elderly	Proportion of Need Currently Met (%)
domiciliary nursing*	25	100
Meals on Wheels*	27	40
laundry service*	20	20
home aid**	28	10
occupational therapy	18	15
physiotherapy	27	70
chiropody	115	70
social day care	17	20
day ward care	4	10

* services needed at least weekly
** services needed at least once very two weeks

Source: Management Services and Research Unit, Department of Health. "Accommodation and Service Needs of the Elderly." Special Report Series No. 46, Wellington, New Zealand, 1976, p. 86. Used by permission.

TABLE 9–1. Assessed Need for, and Provision of, Domiciliary and Other Social Services for the New Zealand Population Aged 65 and Over, 1976

10

The Level of Effort: Quantitative and Qualitative Indicators

The level of effort in providing elderservices varies greatly. Just as needs assessment is an art in its infancy, so is the related problem of measuring the quantity and quality of service provision in relation to the population at risk.

From one point of view, this may be viewed as a management problem, to be tackled by defining objectives and collecting data for the computer from a management information system. In a more fundamental way, it is a conceptual problem, due to the lack of a chronic care model and difficulties in defining what a service is.

Our objective is to assess the stage of development of a service system, national or local, and to be able to measure progress (or lack of it) from a previous baseline. One method we have discussed is to take the index of incapacity/planning guidelines route, as in the New Zealand study, calculating the ratio of helpers per 100,000 population, or 1,000 elderly. For example, in Britain the Department of Health and Social Services called on local authority social services departments to submit ten-year development plans for the period 1973 to 1983; the suggested goal for home helps was about 150 per 100,000 total population, or 12 per 1,000 elderly (DHSS, 35/72, 1972).

This kind of ratio may also be used as a measure of the quantitative coverage achieved in a given year or time frame. Some data are available for cross-national comparisons. For example, Kamerman found that the ratio actually achieved in Britain for the year 1973 was one full-time home help to some 700 total population, by comparison with one to around 260 in Sweden (Kamerman, 1976). Goldberg and Connelly (1978) give more recent figures. For every 1,000 persons aged 65 plus in England in 1976, 87 were receiving home help (compared with 62 in 1970), and the service was, in fact, largely one for the elderly; 87 percent of the 652,800 cases attended in 1976 were 65 plus.

Using data compiled from members' reports to the International Council of Home Help Services, it is possible to get a beginning notion of how the home helper ratio varies in the services reporting. A second indicator, designed to get more accurate measures of full-time equivalence, is the number of work hours per 1,000 population (Table 10–1). Sweden, Norway, and the Netherlands, followed by Britain and Finland, rank highest in numbers of helpers per 100,000 population; for 1977 Norway appears to have exceeded Sweden, whose level of effort may have peaked. Although the data are incomplete, Norway may also have the best ratio of work hours per 1,000.

Other Quantitative Indicators

Other overall measures of effort employed are, for example, the percentage of the Gross National Product devoted to social welfare or, for the elderly population, to social security. Here Wilensky and others have found considerable variance among the 66 countries examined. Looking more closely at the 22 richest countries, Wilensky (1975) found a range in social security spending as a percent of GNP factor costs from 21.0 percent for Austria to 7.9 percent for the United States and 6.2 percent for Japan.

Quantitative indicators used specifically for the aging population include rates of institutionalization and rates of co-residence. Reported rates of placement in long-term care facilities vary and may not be comparable. In 1976, Kamerman reported a range for eight countries from 0.4 percent for Yugoslavia and a little over one percent for Poland to three percent for Britain, five percent for France, Western Germany, and the United States, and nine percent for Canada. The rate is presently estimated to be less than one percent in many developing countries and between 1.5 percent and two percent for Japan. Recently reported data for certain European countries again suggests a broad range, from less than two percent for Hungary, nearly four percent for Austria, and 6.2 percent for Denmark, to about 15 percent for Holland (Amann, 1980).

Variance is also noted in the rate of co-residence of the aged with their adult children or other relatives. According to Sir Ferguson Anderson (1978), it is 10 percent for Sweden, 20 percent for Denmark, 28 percent for the United States, and 42 percent for the United Kingdom. By contrast with other developed countries, Japan has until quite recently boasted of a rate between 70 and 75 percent; this is now declining in Tokyo and other large cities.

Selected Countries	December 1976				
	Total Population (thousands)	Number Home Helpers	Ratio per 100,000 Population	Number Work Hours (thousands)	Ratio per 1,000 Population
Australia*	12,500	60,000	21.97	-	-
Austria	7,525	340	4.5	-	-
Belgium	9,957	8,661	87.0	9,934	998.0
Canada	22,000	3,290	15.0	4,110	510.0
Finland	4,500	6,073	135.0	8,115	1,800.0
France	50,000	7,144	14.3	-	-
West Germany	60,000	12,685	22.0	-	-
Great Britain	49,000	129,724	265.0	-	-
Israel	3,300	350	10.6	300	91.0
Italy	54,000	50	0.1	-	-
Japan	111,934	8,706	7.7	-	-
Netherlands	13,800	82,700	599.0	68,765	5,000.0
Norway	3,988	33,478	840.0	38,135	9,560.0
Sweden	8,220	75,900	923.0	59,000	7,170.0
Switzerland	6,000	2,505	41.7	-	-
U.S.A.	209,000	60,000	28.7	-	-
	December 1977				
Australia*	750	108	14.0	818	11.8
Austria	-	-	-	-	-
Belgium	9,823	9,953	101.0	11,404	1,161.0
Canada	-	-	-	-	-
Finland	4,700	6,943	148.0	9,822	2,089.8
France	53,000	51,062	96.0	32,996	622.5
West Germany	-	-	-	-	-
Great Britain	-	-	-	-	-
Israel	3,500	500	14.0	380	108.5
Italy	-	-	-	-	-
Japan	115,276	11,369	9.8	25,924	217.0
Netherlands	13,500	101,057	748.0	55,924	4,143.0
Norway	4,051	41,184	948.0**	-	-
Sweden	8,200	77,550	946.0	50,700	6,183.0
Switzerland	6,000	3,760	63.0	-	-
U.S.A.	-	-	-	-	-

*Figures for 1977 are for West Australia only
**All but 2,343 of the workers are part-time

Source: Adapted from International Council of Home Help Services, Utrecht, Holland.

TABLE 10–1. Ratio of Home Helpers per 100,000 and Number of Working Hours per 1,000 in Selected Countries, December 1976 and December 1977

Additional countries where the rate of co-residence is reportedly high, although now declining, are Eastern European countries like Yugoslavia and Poland which have severe housing shortages. This is also true in the People's Republic of China where, according to a *New York Times* report, children find it advantageous to live with their parents for many reasons, including the shortage of accommodations and the receipt of old age pensions (Davis-Friedman, 1979, p. 13).

In the absence of other provision for services, a decline in co-residence may indicate less care for the elderly. For example, in Yugoslavia, nearly 70 percent of the old still live in a joint household with one of their children; however, as the young increasingly leave the farm for urban employment, the informal support system has been weakened (Shanas and Sussman, 1977). Also in Greece, where the rate is estimated at about 33 percent, old people are left behind in rural villages where they receive only a meager old age allowance; if their health deteriorates and their children are now urban dwellers, the result is frequently a search for a closed care bed (Amann, 1980).

Likewise, the rate of institutionalization as such indicates little or nothing about the adequacy of the care system. On the one hand, a low ratio of beds might suggest a more substantial effort in domiciliary services, as in the case of Scotland, when compared to the United States (Moore, 1977). On the other hand, the presence of few people in institutions may simply indicate lack of resource allocation to closed care, as in the People's Republic of China.

A more useful indicator would be, therefore, either a ratio of available services to the population at special risk, or measures of actual service delivery such as numbers and percentage of the target population reached. This is often low, as we have seen in the case of Hong Kong. However, this kind of ratio is also low for more developed countries. For example, Meals on Wheels programs serve about one percent of the aged in the United States and Germany and six percent in the United Kingdom (Kamerman, 1976). By contrast, we have noted that in Stockholm the range of open care services offered reaches one out of every three eligible pensioners.

Qualitative Indicators

Qualitative factors may well be as important as quantitative—some would argue *more* important. In fact, there is no sharp dividing line between the two, when elder services are studied; they tend to merge into one another, and are at many points indistinguishable or inseparable. In some cases the use of the word "quality" indicates that no hard data have been collected.

In his analysis of the future of the home help service in the United Kingdom, Moseley (1973) focused primarily on planning ratios, but also gave some attention to the "quality" of the service, by which he meant the range of functions performed, plus accessibility. In the American literature there are numerous references to the three "A's" (accessibility, availability and acceptability) as measures of quality: the medical literature tends rather to stress the "C's" (comprehensiveness, continuity and coordination), which are standards for either an individual case or for the care system in general.

For the United States, the National Council on Homemaker-Home Health Aide Services (now called National HomeCaring Council) has based its certification program on meeting some fourteen basic standards. However, there is an apparent gray area, where one cannot always distinguish the quality of a certified agency (which, by definition, delivers "appropriate" professional services) and the quality of the services themselves. One of their publications includes a glossary which specifies three qualitative elements in service: *intensity*, *duration*, and *complexity*. Intensity means the hours of service in a day and the number of days per week service is provided. Duration means weeks or months, comprising the length of time service is provided. Complexity means the range of (1) homemaker-home health aide tasks, and (2) related health and welfare services (Robinson et al., 1974). Hence the quality of service requires quantitative measures. Efforts are being made both by the National Council and other accrediting bodies, following the leadership of the National League of Nursing, to upgrade their reporting systems, in order to get more information on all of these aspects of service delivery. Meanwhile, reliance is placed on the "quality" of the certified agency.

Additional quality indicators, more related to utilization and consumer satisfaction, would include such things as number of complaints, agency response, and rate of turnover. In order to open up a dialogue in this largely unexplored area, I have made up a list of possible indicators (Table 10–2).

Consumer Satisfaction

Perhaps the most significant qualitative measure is that of consumer satisfaction. In effect, this provides a feedback loop to providers and planners of open care services. As we have seen in Japan and other countries, the needs of older consumers are not necessarily met by available programs. Open care services, like closed care, tend to be oriented more to systems maintenance than to consumer preferences. Even an innovative service, which initially reaches out to the previously rejected, tends to exhibit a kind of Niskanen effect over time. The services offered and the times and places and mode of delivery are geared more to the staff than to client characteristics (Morris and Harris, 1972).

British Home Help Studies

Early British studies of home help generally reported a high degree of consumer satisfaction; this finding may have been related to recipients' fears that the service, always in short supply, might be discontinued if one

Quantitative	Qualitative
number of helpers, full-time	education, training
number of helpers, part-time	skills, orientation
number of supervisors, organizers	qualifications, experience
increase in numbers employed	supervisory pattern
number of working hours	time required for travel, reporting
number of referrals	source (medical, agency, family, self)
average time before service starts	how emergencies handled
24-hour, 7-day coverage: no cases	by whom; what is done
number of cases active	how new referrals handled
percentage of old and old-old	special handling, if any
financial support: sources, amounts	how fund-raising, fee collection handled
number of units of service delivered	consumer satisfaction/dissatisfaction
demographic characteristics of recipients (age, sex, disabled, income)	who find access; who are rejected
functional ratings of recipients	informal support system, functional family
type of housing; location	neighborhood or community support
units of service delivered	services not done
by whom services delivered	trained, paid, supervised
frequency of service	in relation to client need
duration of service	in relation to objectives
condition at termination	as expected, worse, dead
length of waiting list	how waiting list is managed
number of complaints	how agency responds; who handles
client turnover	reasons for dropping out
staff turnover	reasons for dropping out
percentage of eligible population reached	condition of non-recipients

Source: Little, V. C. original.

TABLE 10-2. List of Quantitative and Qualitative Indicators with Special Reference to Home Help Service

were too critical. However, there are clues to support the belief that the system was less than perfect. In basic surveys both Harris (1968) and Hunt (1970) found not only wide local variations in service but also questioned whether service was given for a sufficient number of hours per day and days per week to be effective. Two jobs home helpers do not do—spring-cleaning and window-washing—were both considered very difficult for old people to manage.

Hunt identified three major areas of deficiency: (1) inadequate help for those identified and accepted as being in need; (2) removing help before the recipients could manage on their own; (3) not providing any help at all for others also in need. In addition to the jobs which were never done at all (such as heavy cleaning) were those which were not done on the days the help did not come, such as making fires, beds, and meals.

How did the recipients perceive the service? Most were elderly women, three-fourths of whom had no suggestions for improvement. Those who did complain felt that more time was needed, either more days than twice weekly (generally preferred), or a longer time on the days covered. They also favored a shorter waiting period before service is bugun. A more serious complaint was that home help could be completely withdrawn from one person for a period of time in favor of "needier" cases.

Other British surveys report similar findings. A study for the National Corporation for the Care of Old People (1972) was especially concerned with differences in care given between different types of local authorities. Although county councils had proportionately more help than either country or London boroughs, the latter had both the highest number of cases per home helper and the lowest average number of hours per case. The conclusion was that the home help service is: " . . . good but inadequate . . . it seems to be agreed that 'half a loaf' is better than no bread . . . the trouble is that the half loaf is getting more and more like a few crumbs."

Moseley, by contrast, reviewing his own data from Sunderland (Wales), found the service to be "clearly vital" to the three-quarters of its recipients and "important" to a further ten percent. Moseley also found that clients by and large were satisfied with the frequency, length, and timing of visits which, he concluded are " . . . for areas of average provision broadly correct" (1973).

Messages of dissatisfaction continue to be heard from some elderly recipients. For example, a survey of the opinions of elderly clients referred to the Department of Social Services in the London Borough of Hillingdon found that, of the 25 respondents receiving home help services, 14 were "entirely satisfied," five "quite satisfied," two "had many reservations," and four were "completely dissatisfied." Most people found it "reasonable" to wait up to two weeks for service to begin, while a longer wait was found "unreasonable." Three of the "satisfied" felt, however, that the Department should have responded more quickly to their request and five noted that the home help was not able to come at a regular day and time each week. All of the comments on home help were not quoted in full, but 14 examples were included in the report, seven positive and seven negative (London Borough of Hillingdon, 1974)

An AGE CONCERN survey of the utilization of the health services is of interest because a different group was tapped—597 persons known to local old people's welfare councils. About one-third reported being able to do all housework "easily," another one fourth "with difficulty." The remaining 42 percent all needed help with housework. They reported receiving help as follows: home help, 28 percent; spouse or relative, 16 percent; neighbor or volunteer, 3 percent, and paid domestic help, 4 percent. The AGE CONCERN researchers noted that the percent of their sample receiving home help was high, by comparison with official reports. Some of the quoted comments on the qualitative aspects included: the home helper changes frequently; there is irregularity in the service; two hours weekly is insufficient help for a disabled person; cases in which both a husband and wife are disabled may get no help; and, finally, the expense of domestic or home help fees is a burden for those on fixed incomes (AGE CONCERN on Health, 1972).

The recent complaints about the service sound very much like the same old complaints, perhaps expressed a bit more openly. A review by Goldberg and Connelly (1978) of British research on the home help services is concerned with needs assessment and clients' views of the service, as well as with organization and management problems. Wholly aside from the major issue of lack of equity as between local authorities, which they term "territorial injustice," they conclude that it is impossible to establish an unequivocal relationship between apparent "needs," as indicated by the client's personal capacity and living arrangements, and the amount of service offered. Too many intangibles and complexities are present.

In some five of the local authority studies they reviewed, the amount of help received seemed to depend far more on where the client lived than on his/her circumstances. If this is typical, and if greater horizontal equity is to be achieved, then major resource shifts are necessary which, if feasible at all, can only be done gradually over time.

Seven of the studies reviewed by them explored clients' opinions about the service; only two of these were comprehensive in scope and used representative samples. Both reported a widespread feeling of satisfaction with the service, along with clients' complaints that heavy cleaning and repairs were not done, that there was sometimes uncertainty as to whether the helper would come due to last minute schedule changes, and the like. The same old litany is repeated, suggesting a lack of response on the part of the service. What the researchers recommend is that far more consumer studies be undertaken.

Another clue may surface in an experimental project in Coventry, considered one of the leading British services. The number of home helpers in one district was doubled and an effort made to measure the impact of service saturation on other community services. The result was not the escalation of demand which a few had feared, but rather a steady stream of consumer requests for better service; for the helper to come at more convenient times and more often, to do more of the tasks that the elder person was incapable of doing, and the like.

Summing Up

Surveys of consumer satisfaction, just beginning to be employed, are suspect in many ways. If confined to recipients, they only tap the opinions of people getting the service who, by definition, must like something about it. Other nonrecipient opinions are tapped only rarely, the Japanese studies being one of the first.

In the United States, questions are surfacing about nutrition programs. In the past the Congress has been more generous with funds for food than for social services. However, we are beginning to get clues from recipients and others that meals programs, like the British home help program, are by no means perfect.

A few of the major problems are clear. Attendance at congregate meal sites is as a rule confined to a self-selected group of older people, typically not those in greatest need. Outreach efforts find it difficult to involve the more needy. Menus are planned by a dietician who has to juggle budgetary and nutritional requirements. A beginning effort is now being made to pay attention to ethnic food preferences. As in the case of school lunches, where beets are served to children who don't like them, so broccoli is served to old people whether they eat it or not.

Meals on Wheels programs also have problems. In Hartford, Connecticut, as in Vienna, Austria, there is difficulty in reaching those most in need. Among those reached, there is a high dropout rate because people don't like the food. In any case, a meals service which operates only five days per week fails to solve the problem of eating on the other two days.

The socialization aspects—providing a human contact as well as food—may be overrated. In the inner city, volunteers who make deliveries on their lunch hours don't have time to visit, or fear vandalism to their cars if left unattended. A Texas study found that elders receiving meals by mail were just as enthusiastic as those whose food was delivered in person (*Ageing International,* Aug. 1977).

The Two Faces of Care

These examples suggest a sizable gap between the preferences of older persons and available services. This gap could help explain why so many elderly fail to find access to the system, and why others do not take up their entitlements. In family care, the old lack power and status even when the care is poor. In closed care the resident has little choice but compliance; one who complains too much is labelled a difficult patient and may face staff reprisals, including forced relocation. In open care the older consumer does have another option. He/she may choose not to participate at all or to drop out if the service is unsatisfactory.

In order to gather more evidence, it seems important to follow the Japanese example by going outside the circle of known recipients and studying a comparison group of nonrecipients. Why do they *not* utilize services? Is this due to systemic characteristics, personal preferences which have been insufficiently considered, or other environmental constraints such as location or lack of transportation? How much can be attributed to a mismatch between the needs perceptions of the old and the quantity and quality of what the providers provide?

There is a strong presumption that the small quantity and poor quality of most available services is a major deterrent to greater utilization. A better planned and managed and supported system would help to close the gap between the two faces of care—that which is available on paper, and that which is available in fact.

11

Problems of a
Maturing System:
Beginnings of Service

All over the world there is a mystique about taking the first step in a new service. Any service starts small. It begins with one person with an idea, or a small group. To begin on a voluntary basis was the accepted method in the past, especially in Anglo-Saxon countries. Many charity organizations later evolved into formal agencies with budgets and trained employees (Little, 1975a)

Another traditional method has been for a private agency to experiment with a new mode of delivery, hoping to demonstrate the need and then sell the idea to others. In some countries labor unions have played an important but unacknowledged role in promoting services for their members. The idea is usually not an original one but is borrowed from other countries, or from work with children or the disabled. The first attempt is to provide something which will substitute for care that would normally be done in the home by relatives.

Initial funding comes in various ways, including the proverbial wealthy donor. The American invention of the Community Chest has spread to other countries but not always with the payroll deduction feature: developing countries often prefer to have people put their savings in national provident funds. For private groups all of the well known devices such as food and rummage sales, lotteries, door-to-door canvassing, and getting pledges are always available, along with the more up-to-date walkathons. Finally, it is possible to innovate services in the public sector, whatever the source of the idea, with the necessary administrative backing.

Funding

In our own country the passage of the Older Americans Act in 1965, at a time of high grantsmanship, followed the pattern established for other public programs: a formula for distributing funds through single state agencies, combined with research, demonstration and training grants for approved projects. The demonstration grant still reigns supreme in open care services. When federal grants dry up one falls back on the United Way and on small private foundations.

The defect of the demonstration grant approach is that it has failed to build a service system. Some projects have died, throwing their former clients back into the reject pool. Others stave off their demise by another grant and come to resemble a kind of permanent floating crap game. In addition, a poorly conceptualized, often invisible and underfunded service sector offers few incentives to new entrepreneurs. A lack of creativity appears to be an unintended consequence of funding and cash-flow problems.

Existing providers guard their turfs like the feudal lords of old: traditional agencies, such as family service societies, seem to be fighting for their lives. The gap is being filled by the proprietaries, who are making such strong inroads in home health care that fears are raised that they will take it over, as they have the nursing home industry since 1965. They have shown ability at raising start-up money, hiring personnel, obtaining contracts and, in many cases, at delivering units of service at lower prices. It is the shortage of third-party payment mechanisms which has held their growth down.

Traditional and Modern Approaches

Both in beginning and in continuing a service, there is a contrast between traditional and modern approaches. Like the three components of care, the old and the new may be blended in a unique mix.

The traditional approach is essentially that of providing a family substitute kind of care. Home help, now viewed as the core service for frail elderly, originated as "mother's help," to provide a temporary replacement while the mother was ill or confined. The transfer of this notion to eldercare meant that the helper assumed instead the role of daughter-surrogate, performing tasks which a nearby adult daughter might do. This was seen as requiring little or no training and providing suitable part-time work for women who had their own households and would be willing to work at or close to the minimum wage.

In addition to their assigned tasks, the helpers are not discouraged from doing extras, such as errands, dropping by on weekends, and the like. Thus, the transference/countertransference aspects of the relationship are used in two ways: to ensure the acceptability of the helper as a person entering the home and to get a great deal of family-type services at a low price.

The older model still prevails in a majority of countries. It is largely responsible for the weak image of the service, as evidenced by difficulty in agreeing on a common name to call it. Is it home help, visiting homemaker, home samaritan, *l'aide familiale,* homemaker-home health aide—or some, all, or none of the above? What is it exactly that the helpers do? Here, too, there is lack of agreement. In actuality helpers do innumerable things, not all of which are recorded or reimbursed, and hence do resemble a family more than a bureaucracy. Usually, the major task is seen as housework, especially cleaning up and preparing meals. In England, the helper also does the fires; in Finland the rural helper is expected to help tend the cattle.

Two additional functions are involved: certain kinds of personal care (while drawing the line at professional nursing tasks) and emotional support. It is the third which is especially hard to pinpoint, although most observers are convinced that it is an ingredient. According to one Japanese expert, housekeeping is overreported and counselling underreported.

How the time is divided among various functions is seldom studied. There is little monitoring of what the helper actually does in the allotted time. What attracts people to this line of work? Again, the evidence is sparse, but suggests some desire to be a helping person, get out of the house, earn extra money. When the service was first started in Japan, it initially attracted a superior group of workers, with education and previous experience beyond that found elsewhere. In urban centers in developed countries it is more likely to be a trade-off with equally low-paid aide service in nursing homes.

These largely unexamined personnel issues are looming larger, as the past pool of marginal female labor appears to be drying up. All over the world women's labor force participation is rising, that of middle-aged women most of all. With a foothold in better paying occupations, some with a career ladder and fringe benefits, middle-aged women now have other options of work. Who then is available for the home help tasks? We have seen in Sweden experimentation with other service delivery methods: for example, the specially equipped vans to do heavy work and supply mobile services; the rural postmen to do surveillance and related tasks.

The West European Training Model

The major breakthrough, however, has been the development by Western European countries of a new training model. Originating in Frankfurt, West Germany, this model has spread to France, Switzerland, and the Netherlands. Instead of untrained middle-aged women, secondary school graduates are recruited to the "profession" of home help. The successful applicants are admitted to a training course, which varies in length from one to two years and includes both classroom and practicum learning under supervision. In many ways the course of study resembles a combination of social work and home economics. At the conclusion of the training the graduates are employed either by public agencies or by private agencies receiving government subsidies, as in Holland. The model program in Frankfurt has the practice of continuing to meet with its graduates on a monthly basis for case consultation (Homehelp Services report, Frankfurt seminar, 1975; Council of Europe report, Strasbourg, 1976).

This kind of training is being watched with interest by countries like Britain and Sweden, where the helpers and organizers have in the past had little formal training. It permits a different management strategy in allocating scarce resources. Traditional services tend to work with chronic cases over long periods of time, until death or institutionalization. The result is a skewing of service in favor of known cases. One of the British home help studies, which reported that all cases were underserved in terms of assessed need, also reported a tendency to add services to present cases rather than take on new ones.

By contrast, the European training model calls for a goal-oriented, time limited period of service, ideally six weeks, during which period the professional helper deals with the immediate crisis and mobilizes other support systems before going on to the next assignment. Although some cases have to be carried for longer periods, the management-by-objectives approach is very different from the old fashioned methods. We can see again the contrast between familial and bureaucratic service. This contrast extends from the key manpower issues (who does the work? who trains? who supervises?) to every aspect of the organization and delivery of services (Table 11–1).

Functions of a Mature System

As modern approaches modify the traditional family-substitute approach, additional functions are added to the simple cluster of direct services with which one starts. Most of the added functions are indirect (rather than the laying on of hands), and are often separated from actual service delivery. The multiple functions of a mature care system are outlined in Table 11–2. In performing these functions, management has to take into account all of the parameters listed in our summary of traditional and modern approaches. Administrative decisions are made on the age and gender of the helper, training, supervision, needs assessments, duration and intensity of cases, and populations to be served, as well as on the more mundane aspects of office arrangements and bookkeeping. Hence a mature service

		Traditional	Modern
Name	-	"home help" or variant	"profession" of home help
Tasks	-	housekeeping, personal care, support	counseling, client education, mobilizing community resources
Personnel	-	warm, friendly, middle-aged women, untrained part-time	young trained female, some male full-time
Pay	-	minimum wage, no benefits	established pay scale, fringes
Advancement	-	no career ladder	career ladder
Training	-	none, brief orientation	1-to-2-year certificate program
Supervision	-	minimal, largely administrative supervisors not trained	by professional (nurse, social worker, or team)
Needs assessment	-	by home help organizer	professional team
Administration	-	by organizer	by professional administrator
Nature of case	-	chronic, long-term	short-term, management by objectives
Linkages	-	local government, social work district nurse (occasional)	welfare office, health visitors, general practitioners, housing authority, other community services
Populations served	-	predominantly elderly, some families, means-tested	according to need, multi-problem families, not for the poor alone

Source: Little, V. C. original.

TABLE 11–1. Traditional and Modern Approaches to Home Help

tends to resemble a business in its managerial aspects, while striving to retain the person-focused quality of a caring family.

Case Management

Open care in the community is, therefore, far more complex than closed care in institutions. In closed care all residents are housed under one roof, have an assigned bed, and receive whatever services are provided; payment is usually from a single funding source. In open care, by contrast, the aging individual typically requires a package of services from a variety of providers, each with different funding. When this is combined, as in the United States, with fragmentation and gaps, there is a major problem of

1.	access	single/multiple points of entry; pathways to service
2.	information and referral	information on what? referral to whom? follow-up?
3.	screening/intake	screen out inappropriate and ineligible; distinguish those who want only a single service from multiple service users
4.	assessment and service plan	assessment of the whole person, frequently by multi-disciplinary team; usually includes a home visit and evaluation of relative stress. Review of plan with client and family, modify
5.	purchase of service	requires detailed contracts with providers on amount of service, definition of units, fees, records, vouchers, etc.
6.	delivery of service	by providers
7.	case management	putting together a package of services, monitoring, etc.
8.	advocacy	for more services, more accessible, available and acceptable
9.	reporting	detailed data, including client feedback; MIS (computerized)
10.	funding	pooling funds from federal, state, local, private, third party, fees, etc.
11.	budgeting	program budgeting, 3-yr. forward planning, core budget
12.	planning	begins with older people; must meet government regulations
13.	coordination	much talked of, but seldom seen; major problem of meshing medical, social, environmental and other services on five levels
14.	research	on program operations; utilization of other research
15.	training	of necessary personnel, in conjunction with training institutions

Source: Little, V. C. original.

TABLE 11–2. Functions of a Mature Care System

access to service as well as coordination problems on several systemic levels.

To deal with these problems, a technique is being developed known as both "case management" and "service management." The use of two terms suggests a basic ambiguity: what is the manager managing? If it is the individual case, it is in effect an update of "good, old-fashioned casework," along with the additional complexities introduced by purchase-of-service contracts and multiple providers (Little, Case Management—I and II, unpublished).

At the same time the new case manager is seen as a potential systems manager, monitoring service delivery, pooling funding, helping to weed out inefficient providers and the like. Also, a manager should refrain from direct services; for example, if the client wants personal counseling, this should be referred to one of the service agencies.

In the demonstration projects which have tested this concept, there are elements of both, but the casework aspect predominates.

Coordinating Services: The U.S. Experience

One function of the case manager is coordination. In taking a closer look at this we have little data and few studies to guide us. Those who have begun to study it seem to prefer an interorganizational framework. Earlier, Reid (1964) presented a theoretical approach to interorganizational coordination in social welfare, stressing the facilitation of interdependence. In a similar manner Jones (1975) viewed coordination theoretically as an exchange of resources, to be analyzed in the context of an agency's interorganizational field and its task environment. Davidson (1976) likewise preferred to analyze the planning and coordination of social services in multiorganizational contexts, and proposed a three-stage planning framework. As a case study, he described a demonstration project in which the agencies involved achieved little coordination until faced with the necessity of continuing the program with their own resources. In the most recent major study Gilbert and Specht (1977) focused on the characteristics of model cities.

The conventional wisdom that better coordination of existing services may in and of itself fill the services gap needs to be fully tested in different settings. The most thoroughgoing testing so far is that reported by Aiken and associates (1975), who studied five different demonstration projects aimed at coordinating services for the mentally retarded. The research team found all projects ineffective and proposed an "ideal" tripartite structure; however, the team did not agree as to whether a fully integrated or a decentralized model would be more effective in mobilizing the necessary community support systems.

What Is Coordination?

Jones's definition of coordination has the advantage of parsimony: "the process of combining or relating different services across agency and program lines." The Aiken definition is more sweeping: "the articulation of elements in a social service delivery system so that comprehensiveness of, compatibility among, and cooperation among elements are maximized." In addition to the three parameters of comprehensiveness, compatability and cooperation, the Aiken group found that, to achieve a fully integrated service system, at least four key elements had to be coordinated: program and services, resources, clients, and information. True integration is thus the product of perfect coordination (and was achieved by none of the projects they studied in depth).

In view of present gaps in services, and the fact that we do not yet have a system of services for older people, I will utilize the Jones definition. This assumes the continued existence of many separate service units in a pluralistic society.

Problems of Administrative Coordination, Horizontal and Vertical

In an earlier paper on this subject, I suggested that there were problems of *administrative* coordination horizontally, on the federal level, as well as vertically, from the top down and the bottom up (Little, 1976b). For example, the Federal Council on Aging recommended in its 1975 Annual Report more coordination of three sorts: (1) Title XX and Title III social services planning; (2) coordination between and among federal departments and agencies, both HEW and non-HEW; and (3) coordination of research, demonstration, and evaluation planning and funding. Although 16 or more interagency agreements were supposedly reached at the Washington level, these have not always or often been matched on the state and local levels.

Lack of administrative coordination compounds the difficulties of service coordination at the community level. The Older Americans Act contains a basic ambiguity as to whether to proceed from the top down or from the bottom up. Ideally, planning should begin at the grass roots, with input from older persons, and then proceed upward in an ever-widening stream. In practice, the direction of the flow is the reverse. Regulations and guidelines and funds filter down from Washington to regional offices to state agencies and finally to area planning groups in an ever-increasing flow of paper. In their short lifetime since the 1973 amendments, area agencies have had neither time nor staff to develop their potential coordinating capacities.

More than half of the states and a few cities, such as New York, have sought better coordination by the device of creating super or umbrella agencies for human resources or human services administration. Whatever the merit of the concept, the track record of super agencies is weak. To use two New England states as examples, Connecticut went ahead with an

administrative consolidation of state agencies as promising both economy
and efficiency while Vermont, having tried it, saw the super agency as
adding an extra administrative layer which cost more money and weakened
services.

Five Levels of Service Coordination

In practice it is not always possible to separate administrative coordination
of various governmental units from service coordination. It is important to
do so conceptually, however, in analyzing elderservices. Governmental
units may engage in activities of various kinds, sometimes loosely described as services, but they are not providers of the direct services which
their dollars buy.

As I see it, there are five possible levels of service coordination:

1. *ad hoc* coordination, by telephone or occasional case conference;
2. case management in a purchase-of-service system;
3. program coordination, both within an agency and with others;
4. interagency coordination, involving different services;
5. planned coordination of services.

There is a natural progression in this ordering, from smaller to larger
systems and from smaller to larger territories.

The first level is the traditional casework level. It is still essential and
may be practiced by both social and health agencies, who are also more
inclined to talk with one another. For example, after 1965 it was to the
mutual advantage of visiting nurses' associations and homemaker agencies
to share cases; in fact, it was essential for the latter to do so, in order to get
reimbursement under Titles XVIII and XIX. The picture is changing, as
nursing agencies themselves now provide homemaker/home health aide
services, aiming at self-coordination by more direct control of resources,
rather than exchange.

The second level, case management, stems from current reliance on
purchase-of-service contracts, dating from the 1962 amendments to the
Social Security Act. An elderly client may receive multiple services,
supplied by different providers under contract with a lead agency. For its
part, the lead agency provides a point of access to the system, an assessment mechanism, and a service plan which in turn requires case management.

The third level, program coordination, is difficult to achieve, whether
in a multi-service agency or senior center, and may be the ultimate test of
the personal qualities and management skills of the administrator. For
example, a traditional agency which offers homemaker, Meals on Wheels,

and chore-companion services, tends to administer them as three separate departments, to which different groups of workers and clients are attached. Internal coordination, like external coordination, does not occur easily and requires input.

Program coordination with other agencies will not occur at all, if Aiken and Davidson are correct, unless some kind of power or influence or funding requirement exists. There are signs that in the private sector the United Way is beginning to utilize its revised service identification system (UWASIS), along with planned program budgeting, to move agencies in a coordinating direction. In the public sector there is potential for using the threat of withholding all or part of some federal and state grants to enforce greater program coordination, although this threat is seldom employed. The providers of scarce and expensive services always seem to have the upper hand.

Since service programs for the aged may be located either in a single agency or in separate agencies, or both, the third and fourth levels of coordination overlap to a certain extent. Focusing again on the multiproblem frail elderly client, he/she is faced initially with the problem of access, for which the popular solution has come to be a single entry case management model. However, where tried, this approach has proved expensive both in start-up and operation; it succeeds in serving only a small percentage of the eligible population. Hence, other kinds of interagency arrangements must be sought. Influence alone will not suffice; it needs to be supplemented by interagency agreements and daily monitoring and, above all, subsidized transportation for clients. If the client is not transported, the service itself must travel.

Voluntary coordination among providers seldom occurs. A provider has difficulty in managing his own cash flow and related problems, much less those of his peers. Any provider is engaged in systems maintenance and tends to favor his own services. In some instances, a merger of agencies may occur under duress, because of funding problems. For example, homemaker agencies in the Northeast are being forced either to give up the service or to merge with visiting nurses. This changes the focus of the coordinating problem but not its nature.

The fifth level, planning coordination, can, as suggested, be implemented to a degree in the private sector, as United Ways grapple more effectively with budgetary planning. In the public sector, Title XX, in spite of a weak start in many states, also has this potential. Services for the elderly, omitted or given minor attention in the first year of planning, are now receiving greater attention.

When state offices of aging are able to make more input to the Title XX planning agency, there is improvement. Few states, however, have looked beyond the paper planning process to actual services coordination.

Models of Service Coordination

My studies of demonstration projects in the United States found that the relative amount of success achieved at the five different levels of coordination varied with the individual project and its leadership, but more importantly with the central thrust of the program. I used a fourfold classification: *medical, social services, mixed socio-medical,* and *mediating. Medical* includes hospital-based home care, community nursing agencies and variants, such as hospitals without walls. *Social services* includes the Massachusetts statewide system of local home care corporations, the three Midwest community systems described by Simpson and Farrow (1973), and the now defunct Personal Care Project in Hartford, Connecticut. *Mixed socio-medical* includes such projects as Minneapolis Age and Opportunities Center, Inc., On Lok and Project 222 in San Francisco. *Mediating* includes housing projects, mayors' commissions and area agencies on aging.

Table 11–3 presents, in schematic form, my impressions of the extent to which the projects I have studied coordinate services for the elderly on the five levels. How much coordination are we willing to pay for? Coordination by whom? Is perfect coordination either possible or desirable? In trying to answer these questions we may look to the experience of other countries.

Coordination in Other Countries

In countries lacking a formal structure of open care services, the family is used both to provide services, to find needed outside help (in particular, medical), and to do whatever coordinating is done. The traditional coordinating device has been for the housewife to stay home. If the family doesn't do it, the women's committees and other informal supports are available as a backup, as in Western Samoa. In countries with a public welfare service base, the local welfare office becomes the focal point for both case and service management. The task is more complex where the private sector delivers services under subsidy, contract or other method of payment. Who coordinates? The public agency retains fiscal control but is seldom in a position to do more than monitor service delivery *ex post facto*. There is a gap to be filled, or left unfilled. How is this done elsewhere?

American students of Britain have different attitudes toward the British system and its success in coordinating as well as delivering services. The majority take the point of view that Britain is a "caring society," which does a far better job than we do. Austin (1976) depicted well-marked pathways for help with the elderly, permitting the meshing of medical,

Models	Level 1 ad hoc	Level 2 Case Mgt.	Level 3 Program	Level 4 Inter-ag.	Level 5 Planning
Medical					
a. home care	m	0	0	m	0
b. comm. nurs.	x	0	x	x	0
Social Services					
Midwest*					
St. Paul	x	0	x	x	x
Inkster	x	0	x	m	x
Delta-Menom.	x	x	x	0	x
Mass. Home Care	x	x	0	b	b
Pers. Care Proj.	x	x (s.wk.)	0	0	0
Mixed					
Triage (Conn.)	x	x (n.pr.)	0	0	0
M.A.O.	x	x (team)	x	x	m
On Lok	x	x (team)	x	b	b
222	x	0	b	b	x
Mediating					
Housing	x	0	0	0	0
Mayor's Comm.	x	0	0	0	b
AAA's	x	0	0	0	b

*
as described by Simpson & Farrow   Key: x = present
                                            0 = absent
                                            m = minimal
                                            b = beginning

Source: Little, V. C. original.

TABLE 11–3. Extent to Which Existing Models Coordinate Services for the Elderly on Five Levels

social, and housing provisions. Schneidermann, on the other hand, took a minority position, finding difficulties of collaboration between the health and social services sectors, largely because they operate under different administrative structures (1978).

As Schneidermann points out, the fact that there are two discrete organizations that are funded and administered at different levels of government results in a lack of congruence, structurally, organizationally, fiscally, and politically. This poses real problems in providing residential care for the aged and chronically ill, a group of patients who fall between the cracks and "appear to be outcasts in the system." Direct professional contact between physicians and social workers is weak, because it often involves persons who differ substantially in age, experience, and degree of specialization. So coordination fails to happen.

My own observations in Britain have convinced me that there is truth in both the majority and minority views. I know of notable examples of collaboration between district nurses, social workers and home help organizers, as well as failures. The role of the health visitor appears to be a way of bridging the gap and effecting better collaboration with physicians. Highly trained clinical social workers, with a good background in psychiatry and other skills, apparently do not have the communications problem which the less trained generic worker may experience.

Turning from Britain to Sweden, I commented earlier on the apparent tension there between the social services and the medical sectors. As in Britain, the two are under different administrative structures, with medical/health at the county level. Again, examples could be cited both of good collaboration and of difficulties in communicating adequately about certain kinds of cases. After reviewing additional material from Sweden, I have come to a somewhat different point of view, that the separation of the two systems under discrete administrative auspices may have its advantages, as well as disadvantages, for eldercare. If the two agree on which persons are to be allocated to which sector and who is to take primary responsibility, there is no problem. However, the borderline or gray area of mixed cases remains. To the extent that service houses are able to fulfill their initial promise and maintain severely disabled pensioners in open care, there will be fewer cases which fall through the cracks.

The European Centre for Social Welfare Training and Research is interested in the coordination issue, as well as in open care, and has already had discussions of beginning projects in countries as diverse as Britain, The Netherlands and Canada, focused mainly on various kinds of team work.

In Japan, whose service system was copied from Britain and Sweden, the question of coordination is differently viewed. Case coordination is the job of the social worker for the aged in the local welfare office, along with supervision of the home helpers. Because the service is funded one-third each from three different levels of government (central, provincial and local), the problem presents as one of securing intergovernmental fiscal coordination.

In Hong Kong, as in Singapore, there is a coordinating mechanism for the private sector, in the form of a Council of Social Service. In each case the Council occupies a building which also houses the head offices of member agencies; apparently, co-location increases the chances of collaboration. In addition, the Councils see themselves as the counterpart of government; as such, they participate in official planning and program coordinating efforts. Co-location may not be the final answer, but there is an advantage to the private sector in presenting a united front to the controllers of the public pursestrings.

Over- and Underutilization

Problems of access to and availability of elderservices often result in underutilization. According to Gates (1980), services are simultaneously both over- and underutilized. He distinguishes four subsets of the total population: (1) the segment which is found to need and also demands services: (2) the subset which does not fall within the defined criteria for need, but which demands or utilizes the services; (3) the subset which falls within the criteria of need, but does not demand them; (4) the portion which neither needs nor demands services.

What is the present situation? A look at escalating health expenditures suggests an overutilization of reimbursed hospital/medical care and nursing home care, with an underutilization of open care. Health care utilization studies are beginning to find evidence of what are called "outliers," or heavy users, who both need and demand a disproportionate share of scarce services. Thus subset (1) is served at the expense of subset (3). If open care services were larger in quantity, better in quality and better located, there could be an improved utilization rate for subset (3). However, according to Gates, there are no perfect solutions for the access problem.

Not accessing the service system is also a basic human right, along with access. Older persons have the same right of self-determination and of choice from among available options as younger persons. Our concern is to present them with valid options in the form of an accessible, available, and acceptable open care system.

12

Summary and Conclusions: Trends and Innovations in Elderservices

There appears to be a bad fit between aging, industrialization, and modernization. With industrialization more people live to advanced ages and experience a longer period of retirement. With modernization there is a rising level of expectation as to the quality of life to be shared by all members of the society, including the old.

Certain values are universal: that the old should stay in the community as long as possible, that there is intergenerational reciprocity, and that families care. An emerging value is that the old, like people of all ages, should have genuine options or choice positions.

Open care is such an option but continues to play the Cinderella role. All over the world, regardless of ideology and political system, open care is less developed and less funded than closed. Although societies are at different stages of development, there is none which is fully satisfied with its care system. The four we have examined in depth (Western Samoa, Hong Kong, Japan, and Sweden) have their own mix of open, closed, and unorganized care. Developing and developed societies can both learn lessons from one another in achieving a better mix in the area of long-term care.

There is evidence of social learning, certainly by the Japanese and Hong Kong leaders, as well as considerable interchange and imitation among Western European countries. Britain and the United States are somewhat involved with one another and are beginning to interact more with Western Europe. Asian developments, on the whole, have received less attention from Western students, with the exception of Japan.

Each country has its devices and its innovations which are new to itself, if not always to others. On balance, however, the number of innovations in service design and delivery is surprisingly small. The rural postman in Sweden has been copied in Norway, Britain, West Germany and elsewhere. Home help as the core service continues to experience accretions, deletion and reorientation. By and large most elderservices are conceptualized as family substitutes and are frequently copied from services for children.

Some of the services in a developed country are needed because of deficits in other systems, for example, transportation in the United States. Others are needed because of the dysfunctionalities of legislated programs, for example, helping older people fill out the necessary forms and produce the documentation needed to establish eligibility. This is one of the unintended consequences produced by a variety of bureaucratic structures.

The weak conceptualization of community services is reflected both in a larger investment in closed care and in the considerable variance of effort. Because open care is weak, the unorganized care sector in most countries provides the bulk of the services which old people receive, about 80 percent in the United States. Hence, greater resource allocation to family backup and respite services is recommended, in the form of financial payments, income tax relief, housing subsidies, medical support, month-in-month-out hospitalization, family vacations and the like. These kinds of measures are taken in Sweden, Britain, Japan and elsewhere and deserve a wider application.

Present delivery of services is shown to be inadequate, both quantitatively and qualitatively. In some communities it is also largely invisible and unknown, in spite of such efforts as information and referral and outreach. It is mysterious to planners and decisionmakers as well because of the inadequate data base even in Level 4 systems.

It is hard for us to explain why so many older Americans fail to find access to the system, or drop out, or fall through the net. I have used the expression "two faces of care" to describe the common situation: services which exist on paper and do not exist in fact for a particular older person at a given place and time. "Territorial injustice" is just one kind of inequity experienced by those with unmet service needs.

Insufficient attention has been paid to the locus of services and to the question of whether they are "individual" or "collective," to use the Swedish terminology. Tobin et al. (1977) have made a similar distinction between "home-delivered" and "congregate-delivered" services; the latter include not only congregate residence (that is to say, closed care), but also congregate-organized, such as senior centers, nutrition sites and outpatient medical care.

As we have noted, there is a major problem in transporting disabled individuals to congregate sites and other destinations. In the United States we have tried a number of ingenious, albeit expensive, devices, such as specially fitted buses and vans, Dial-A-Ride, and the like. Still much transportation is done by relatives, with taxis and ambulances reserved for emergencies. Escorts are often required and the current supply of volunteers is low. The option is to have the service delivered to the home on an individual case basis. The higher the rate of hourly pay of the service deliverer, the more costly in budgetary terms.

Another approach to providing a desirable kind of congregate residence with built-in services is that of the Swedish service houses and, to a lesser extent, the Hong Kong hostels. As the resident population ages and becomes more frail, more services are required.

In our own country it is now more possible for churches and other nonprofit groups, as well as towns and municipalities, to utilize available HUD (Housing and Urban Development) funds for special elderly housing, with services. In addition to money, there are two other major requirements: (1) a specially designed building and environment; and (2) services on the premises with staff. Once more, it is easier for the average person to conceptualize the need for the structure than the need for built-in services.

Another approach, being tried in Israel, stems from a pessimistic estimate of the possibilities of greatly expanding community services. Where will the funding come from? At the same time they have already demonstrated the feasibility of deinstitutionalizing older patients and returning them to community living (Bergman, 1973). Out of this has grown the concept, embodied in the current Israeli ten-year development plan for the aging, of remodeling existing institutions, and training their staffs to look "outward" beyond their walls and also serve community residents. This would promote continuity of care, should hospitalization be required, and would also facilitate the return to community living. The implementation of the concept requires developing additional institutions in regions now underserved and adding a ring of satellites to both old and new facilities. To base open care in closed care and somehow involve the unorganized care sector may be one answer.

References and Suggested Readings

References and Suggested Readings

For the convenience of readers, references to works cited in the four country chapters (Western Samoa, Hong Kong, Japan, and Sweden) are listed separately.

AGE CONCERN on Health. Discussion Document No. 3. London: AGE CONCERN—England, March 1972.

Ageing International: Information bulletin of the International Federation on Ageing, August 1977, 7.

Aiken, Michael et al. *Coordinating human services*. San Francisco: Jossey-Bass, 1975.

Amann, Anton. *Open care for the elderly in seven European countries*: A pilot study in the possibility and limits of care. London: Pergamon Press, 1980.

Anderson, Sir F. Lecture delivered at Post-Conference International Symposium on Ageing, Kyoto, Japan, August 1978.

Anderson, W. F. Prevention aspects of geriatric medicine. *Journal of the American Geriatrics Society*, 1974, *22*, 385–392.

Austin, M. J. A network of help for England's elderly. *Social Work*, March 1976, 114–119.

Avant, W. P. & Dressel, P. L. Comparative perceptions of the needs of the elderly and their implications for service delivery: An analysis of a metropolitan community. Paper presented at the 29th Annual Meeting of the U.S. Gerontological Society, New York, New York, October 1976.

Bergman, S. Facilitating living conditions for aged in the community. *Gerontologist*, Summer 1973, 184–188.

Berkman, B. G. & Rehr, H. Social needs of the hospitalized elderly: A classification. *Social Work*, July 1972, *17*, 4, 80–89.

Binstock, R. & Shanas, E. (Eds.) *Handbook of aging and the social sciences*. New York: Van Nostrand Reinhold, 1976.

Branch, L. *Understanding the health and social service needs of people over 65*. Boston: University of Mass., Center for Survey Research, 1977.

Cantor, M. H. & Johnson, J. L. The informal support system of the "familyless" elder—who takes over? Paper presented at the 31st Annual Meeting of the U.S. Gerontological Society, Dallas, Texas, November 1978.

Churchman, C. W. *The systems approach*. New York: Dell, 1968.

Comptroller-General of the U.S. *Report to the Congress*. Home health—the need for a national policy to better provide for the elderly. Washington, D.C.: Gov't Printing Office, Dec. 30, 1977. (HRD-78-19).

Council of Europe. *Social cooperation in Europe: "Home help services."* Strasbourg, 1976.

Cowgill, D. O. & Holmes, Lowell D. *Aging and modernization*. New York: Appleton-Century-Crofts, 1972.

Davidson, S. M. Planning and coordination of social services in multi-organizational contexts. *Social Service Review*, March 1976, 117–137.

Davis-Friedman, D. quoted by Fox Butterfield. *New York Times*, July 29, 1979, 13.

Department of Health and Social Security (England). Social authority social services 10-year development plans, 1973–1983. Circular 35/72, 31 August 1972.

Dependency of the elderly in New York City. Report of a Research Utilization Workshop. Community Council of Greater New York, October 1978.

Doherty, N. J. C. & Hicks, B. C. The use of cost-effectiveness analysis in geriatric day care. *Gerontologist*, October 1975, *15*, 412–417.

Fisher, D. H. *Growing old in America*. New York: Oxford University Press, 1977.

Gates, B. L. *Social program administration: The implementation of social policy*. Englewood Cliffs, N.J.: Prentice-Hall, 1980.

Gilbert, N. & Specht, H. *Coordinating social services: An analysis of community, organizational and staff characteristics*. New York: Praeger, 1977.

Gilbert, N. & Specht, H. *Dimensions of social welfare policy*. Englewood Cliffs, N.J.: Prentice-Hall, 1974.

Goldberg, E. M. & Connelly, N. Home help services for the elderly: A review of recent research. London: Center for Policy Studies, 1978 (mimeo.).

Gurland, B. et al. Assessing the older person in the community: Findings and experiences from a cross-national study. *International Journal of Aging and Human Development*, 1977–1978, 7, 4 & 8, 1.

Harris, A. T. assisted by Clausen, R. *Social welfare for the elderly: A study in thirteen local authority areas in England, Wales, and Scotland*. London: (HMSO), 1968, Government Social Survey.

Harris, L. & associates. *The myth and reality of aging in America*. Washington, D.C.: National Council on the Aging, 1975.

Homehelp services, where they are and where they are going. Report of the Second International Homehelp Seminar, Frankfurt, West Germany, April 1975.

Hunt, A. assisted by Fox, J. *The home help service in England and Wales*. London: (HMSO), 1970. Government Social Survey.

Isaacs, B., M.D. & Neville, Y. *The measurement of need in old people*. Edinburgh: Scottish Home and Health Dept., 1976.

Jones, T. Some thoughts on coordination of services. *Social Work*, September 1975, 375–378.

Kahana, E. Service needs of urban aged. Paper presented at the 27th Annual Meeting of the U.S. Gerontological Society, Portland, Oregon, October 1974.

Kahana, E. & Fairchild, T. Dimensions of service need among urban aged. Paper presented at the 29th Annual Meeting of the U.S. Gerontological Society, New York, New York, October 1976.

Kahn, A. & Kamerman, S. *Not for the poor alone*. Philadelphia: Temple University Press, 1975.

Kahn, A. & Kamerman, S. *Social services in international perspective*. Washington, D.C.: (GPO) circa 1977. HEW/SRS 76-05704.

Kamerman, S. B. Community services for the aged: The view from eight countries. *Gerontologist*, 1976, *16*, 6, 529–537.

Kamerman, S. & Kahn, A. *Social services in the United States: Policies and programs*. Philadelphia: Temple University Press, 1976.

Kendig, H. L., Jr. & Warren, R. The adequacy of census data in planning and advocacy for the elderly. *Gerontologist*, 1976, *16*, 5, 392–397.

Laslett, P. *Household and family in past time*. London: Cambridge University Press, 1972.

Little, V. C. Assessing the needs of the elderly: State of the art. *International Journal of Aging and Human Development*, 1980–1981, *11*, 1, 67–78.

Little, V. C. For the elderly: An overview of services in industrially developed and developing countries. In *Reaching the aged*: Social services in forty-four countries. Social Service Delivery Systems: An International Annual, Vol. 4, Teicher, M. I., Thursz, D. & Vigilante, J. (Eds.). Belmont, Calif.: Sage, 1979, 149–173.(a)

Little, V. C. Open care for the aging: Alternate approaches. *Aging*, November-December 1979 (International Issue), *301–302*, 10–24.(b)

Little, V. C. Open care for the aged: Swedish model. *Social Work*, July 1978, *23*, 4, 272–278.

Little, V. C. Planning and delivering elderly services: The Hong Kong experience. *Hong Kong Journal of Social Work*, Fall 1979, 2–9.(c)

Little, V. C. in Nusberg, C. (Ed.) Home help services for the aging around the world. Washington, D.C.: International Federation on Ageing, 1975, 16–23, 22–26, 32–43.(a)

Little, V. C. Aging in Western Samoa. Paper presented at the 29th Annual Meeting of the U.S. Gerontological Society, New York, New York, October 1976.(a)

Little, V. C. Case Management, I and II. Unpublished manuscripts.

Little, V. C. A comparison of the impact and effect of home help services in Japan and homemaker-home health aide services in the United States. Paper presented at the XIth International Congress of Gerontology, Tokyo, Japan, August 1978.

Little, V. C. Social services for the elderly: With special attention to Asia and the West Pacific region. Paper presented at the 27th Annual Meeting of the U.S. Gerontological Society, Portland, Oregon, October 1974.

Little, V. C. Coordinating services for the elderly. Paper presented at the Governor's Bicentennial Conference, Honolulu, 1976. (Rev. version, 1977).(b)

Little, V. C. Factors influencing the provision of in-home services in developed and developing countries. Paper presented at the Xth International Congress of Gerontology, Jerusalem, Israel, 1975.(b)

London Borough of Hillingdon, Social Services Dept. Client opinions. In University of Birmingham (England), Clearing House for Local Authority Social Services Research, 1974, *1*, 31–40.

Lurie, E. Limits to informal support systems of the elderly. Paper presented at the Annual Meeting of the Western Gerontological Society, San Francisco, May 1979.

Mahoney, K. The elderly and valued community services: A predictive model. Prizewinning student paper, U.S. Gerontological Society, New York City, October 1976.

Mahoney, K. A national perspective on community differences in the interaction of the aged with their adult children. Paper read at the 30th Annual Meeting of the U.S. Gerontological Society, San Francisco, Calif., November 1977.

Manchester (England). *Survey of the needs of the elderly,* 1972.

McKain, W. C. (Consultant). *Dignity for the living.* Norwich, Conn.: Area Agency on Aging, 1975.

Monk, A. & Cryns, A. G. Service needs of the rural elderly: A comparative study of agency personnel and public officials. Paper presented at the 29th Annual Meeting of the U.S. Gerontological Society, New York, New York, October 1976.

Monk, A. & Cryns, A. G. The awareness and need for social services: An area study. Paper presented at the 30th Annual Meeting of the U.S. Gerontological Society, Louisville, Ky., October 1975.

Moore, F. New issues for in-home services. *Public Welfare,* Spring 1977, 26–37.

Morris, R. & Harris, E. Home health services in Massachusetts, 1971: Their role in care of the long-term sick. *American Journal of Public Health,* August 1972, *62*, 8, 1088–1092.

Moseley, L. G. The future of the home help service in the United Kingdom. *Zeitschrift fur Gerontologie,* 1973, *6*, 4, 333–341.

Moss, M. S. et al. Needs and difficulties of older persons as perceived by the aged and their families. Paper presented at the International Congress of Gerontology, Jerusalem, Israel, June 1975.(a)

Moss, M. S. et al. Elderly community residents: Is their statement of "wants" reflective of their subsequent acceptance of services? Paper presented at the 30th Annual Meeting of the U.S. Gerontological Society, Louisville, Ky., October 1975.(b)

National Corporation for the Care of Old People. *Services for the elderly at home: A review of current needs and problems.* London: Bedford Square Press, 1972.

Neugarten, B. The future and the young-old. *Gerontologist,* Feb. 1975, *15*, Pt. II, 4–9.

New Zealand. Department of Health, Management Services and Research Unit. *Accommodation and service needs of the elderly.* Special Report Series No. 46. Wellington, New Zealand: A. R. Shearer, 1976.

Nusberg, C. (Ed.). *Ageing in international perspective*. Washington, D.C., International Federation on Ageing, 1979.

Nusberg, C. (Ed.). *Ageing international*. Newsletter.

Nusberg, C. (Ed.). *Home help services for the ageing around the world*. Washington, D.C.: International Federation on Ageing, 1975.

Palmore, E. *The honorable elders: A cross-cultural analysis of aging in Japan*. Durham, N.C.: Duke University Press, 1975.

Project SHARE. Needs assessment. Human Services Bibliography Series No. 2, August 1976.

Province of Manitoba, Department of Health and Social Development; Havens, B., Research Director. *Aging in Manitoba: Needs and resources, 1971*. Winnipeg, Manitoba, 1973.

Reader, G., M.D. Types of geriatric institutions. Paper presented at the IXth International Congress of Gerontology, Kiev, USSR, July 1972; a revised version appears in the *Gerontologist*, Autumn 1973, *13*, 3, 290.

Reid, W. Interagency coordination in developing prevention and control. *Social Service Review*, Dec. 1964, *35*, 4.

Robinson, N. et al. Costs of homemaker-home health aide and alternative forms of service: A survey of the literature. New York: National Council for Homemaker-Home Health Aide Services, Inc., 1974.

Schneidermann, L. Collaboration between the health and social services in England. *Social Work*, May 1978, 192–197.

Services for the elderly at home: A review of current needs and problems. London: Bedford Square Press, 1972. Published for the National Corporation for the Care of Old People.

Shanas, E. The health of older people: A social survey. Cambridge, Mass.: Harvard University Press, 1962.

Shanas, E. et al. Old people in three industrial societies. New York: Atherton, 1968.

Shanas, E. Health status of older people: Cross-national implications. *American Journal of Public Health*, 1974, *64*, 3, 261–264.

Shanas, E. Measuring the home health needs of the aged in five countries. *Journal of Gerontology*, 1971, *26*, 37–40.

Shanas, E. Social myth as hypothesis: The case of the family relations of old people. *Gerontologist*, 1979, *19*, 1, 3–9.

Shanas, E. & Streib, G. (Eds.). *Social structure and the family: Generational relations*. Englewood Cliffs, N.J.: Prentice-Hall, 1965.

Shanas, E. & Sussman, M.B. (Eds.). *Family, bureaucracy, and the elderly*. Durham, N.C.: Duke University Press, 1977.

Silverstone, B. An overview of research on informal supports: Implications for policy and practice. Paper presented at the 31st Annual Meeting of the U.S. Gerontological Society, Dallas, Texas, November 1978.

Simmons, L. W. *The role of the aged in primitive societies*. New Haven: Yale University Press, 1945.

Simpson, D. F. & Farrow, F. G. Three community systems of services to the aging. *Social Casework*, February 1973.

Svane, O. Assessment of needs of care for the elderly. *Zeitschrift fur Gerontologie*, 1973, *6*, 4, 307–315.

Tobin, S. et al. *Effective social services for older Americans*. Detroit: University of Michigan—Wayne State Gerontology Center, 1977.

United Nations reports: Question of the elderly and the aged. Report of the Secretary-General to the General Assembly, A/9126, August 28, 1973. The aging: Trends and policies, Department of Economic and Social Affairs, ST/ESA/22, 1975. Aging: The developed and developing world: A report on recommendations prepared by Walter M. Beatie, Jr., April 3–5, 1978. Aging: Bulletin on Aging, issued by the Social Development branch, Secretariat, 1976.

United Way of Eastern Fairfield County, Human Services Needs Assessment Project. A community assessment of needs within the Greater Bridgeport area, 1977.

Wallach, H. C. The evaluation of social and health delivery systems for the aging: Unobtrusive approaches. In *Gerontology at St. Michael's, 1977*, Winooski, Vt.: St. Michael's College, 1977.

Wethersfield, Conn. *Survey of elderly needs and potentialities*, 1977.

Wilensky, H. *The welfare state and equality*. Berkeley, Calif.: University of California Press, 1975.

Wilensky, H. & Lebeaux, C. N. *Industrial society and social welfare*. New York: Russell Sage, 1967.

Selected references on the four countries studied in depth follow:

Hong Kong

Chow, N. W. S. An appraisal of proposals of the Green Paper on a programme of social security development in Hong Kong. *Hong Kong Journal of Social Work*, 1978, *12*, 1, 20–28.

Hong Kong Council of Social Service. *Report of study of the social service needs of the elderly in Hong Kong*, March 1978,

Hong Kong Council of Social Service. *Welfare Digest*. Newsletter.

Hong Kong, 1979. Official yearbook, Hong Kong Government.

Hong Kong Government: Policy statements. (Available from Government Printer). The five-year plan for social welfare development in Hong Kong, 1973–1978 (1973). Social welfare in Hong Kong: The way ahead (1973). Care in the community: The right basis for services to the elderly: Report of a working party (1973). Social welfare into the 1980's (the White Paper of April, 1979).

Meeting the changing needs of the elderly in Hong Kong. Paper prepared by the Hong Kong Delegation to the XIth International Congress of Gerontology, Tokyo, Japan, August 1978.

Japan

Aoi, K. The meaning of life for Japanese elderly. Paper presented at the XIth International Congress of Gerontology, Tokyo, Japan, August 1978.

Broberg, M., Melching, D. & Maeda, D. Planning for the elderly in Japan. *Gerontologist*, 1975, *15*, 3, 242–247.

Campbell, J. C. Entrepreneurial bureaucrats and programs for old people in Japan. Paper presented at the 1978 Annual Meeting of the American Political Science Association, New York, September 1978.

Dessau, D. (Ed.). *Glimpses of social work in Japan*. (Rev. ed.). Tokyo: Social Workers' International Club of Japan, 1968.

Honma, M., Shimizu, Y. & Maeda, D. Measurement of the needs for home delivery services for the elderly. Paper presented at the XIth International Congress of Gerontology, Tokyo, Japan, August 1978.

Little, V. C. A comparison and evaluation of the impact and effect of home help services in Japan and homemaker-home health aide services in the United States. Paper presented at the XIth International Congress of Gerontology, Tokyo, Japan, August 1978,

Japan Institute for Gerontological Research and Development, *Ageing in Japan*, Tokyo, 1978.

Maeda, D. Innovative services for the elderly in Japan. Paper presented at the Xth International Congress of Gerontology, Jerusalem, Israel 1975.

Maeda, D. et al. *Impaired old people and home help services*. Tokyo Metropolitan Institute of Gerontology, Sociology Department, 1979. (Available only in Japanese language.)

Maeda, N. & Kagawa, K. Studies on the needs and services of day care for the elderly patients in Japan. Report presented at the XIth International Congress of Gerontology, Tokyo, Japan, August 1978.

Palmore, E. *The honorable elders*: A cross-cultural analysis of aging in Japan. Durham, N.C.: Duke University Press, 1975.

Plath, D. Japan: The after years. In Cowgill, D. and Holmes, L. *Aging and modernization*. New York: Appleton-Century-Crofts, 1972.

Shimizu, Y. & Maeda D. et al. Difficulties of the families living with and caring for impaired old people. Paper presented at the XIth International Congress of Gerontology, Tokyo, Japan, August 1978.

Social Welfare Services in Japan. Annual government publication.

Vogel, E. *Japan as number one*: Lessons for America. Cambridge, Mass.: Harvard University Press, 1979.

Sweden

Bengtsson, I., Minister of Labor, 1974–1976. Economic security in old age: Swedish pension models. Paper prepared for Seminars on Facing an Aging Society, U.S.A. and Canada, October 1978.

Bozzetti, L. P., et al. *The aged in Sweden*. I: The country, its people and institu-

tions (Bozzetti, L. P., & Sherman, S.); II: A systems approach—The Swedish
    model (Bozzetti, L. P.); III: The home Samaritans and the marginal elderly
    (Bozzetti, I. L. & Bozzetti, L. P.). *Psychiatric Annals*, 7:3. New York: Insight
    Publishing Co., March 1977.
Elmer, A. Sweden's model system of social services administration. In *Meeting
    human needs: An overview of nine countries*. Social Services Delivery Sys-
    tems, Vol. 1. Beverly Hills, Calif.: Sage, 1975, 196–219.
Kane, R. L. & Kane, R. A. *Long-term care in six countries*. Fogarty International
    Center. Proceedings No. 33; DHEW Publ. No. (NIH) 76–1207. Washington,
    D.C.: GPO, 1976.
Little, V. C. Open care for the aged: Swedish model. *Social Work*, 1978, *23*, 4,
    282–287.
McRae, J. M. Elderly housing in northern Europe. In *Ageing in international
    perspective*. International Federation on Ageing, 1979, 1–9.
Nusberg, C. (Ed.). *Ageing in international perspective*. Washington D.C.: Interna-
    tional Federation on Ageing, 1979. (Includes chapters by McCrae & Little.)
Rosenthal, A. H. *The social programs of Sweden*. Minneapolis: University of
    Minnesota, 1967.
Salzer, E. M. Growing old in Sweden. *Current Sweden 200*, September 1978 (2).
Sidel, V. W. & Sidel, R. *A healthy state: An international perspective on the crisis
    in United States medical care*. New York: Pantheon, 1978.
Sidel, V. W. & Sidel, R. Medical care in Sweden—Planned pluralism. *Social
    change in Sweden 10*, February 1979.
Swedish Institute. Old-age care in Sweden. *Fact Sheets on Sweden*, September
    1978.
Thunberg, T. The Swedish pension scheme. *Current Sweden 148*, January 1977.
Thursz, D. & Vigilante, J. (Eds.). *Meeting human needs: An overview of nine
    countries*. Social Services Delivery Systems, Vol. 1. Beverly Hills, Calif.:
    Sage, 1975.
Von Sydow, T., First Secretary, National Swedish Board of Health and Welfare,
    Stockholm. Home sweet home . . . housing and social services for Swedish
    citizens. Paper prepared for Seminars on Facing an Aging Society, U.S.A. and
    Canada, October 1978.

Western Samoa

Cernak, K. Western Samoa's elderly people. *Pacific Health*, 1979, *12*, 6–9.
Little, V. C. Aging in Western Samoa. Paper presented at the 29th Annual Meeting
    of the U.S. Gerontological Society, New York, New York, October 1976.
Mead, M. *Coming of age in Samoa*. New American Library, Mentor, 1928.
Western Samoa. Department of Economic Development. *Review of the economy*,
    1977. Health Planning and Information Unit, Health Department, *Health
    statistics for Western Samoa, 1977*, 1977.

Index

Index

Community Housing
Choices for Older Americans
M. Powell Lawton, Ph.D. and **Sally Hoover, M.A.,** editors

Discusses the national characteristics of housing and house-holds occupied by the aged, using research findings and active service program data. The authors describe innovative housing programs such as home-sharing, small-unit renovation, and local-area-based service programs that relate to the concept of community-based long-term care. Special attention is paid to the problems of high-need populations, including minorities, rural elderly, and tenants of single-room occupancy hotels.

This volume is the first to integrate the concerns of the housing and social service networks, providing a solid introduction to students of social gerontology, social work, planning, and public administration.

336 pages   hardcover   1981

Aging and the Environment
Theoretical Approaches
M. Powell Lawton, Ph.D., Paul G. Windley, Arch.D., and
Thomas O. Byerts, A.I.A., M.Arch., editors

How should a nursing home be designed in order to encourage social interaction among patients while respecting their need for privacy? What psychological needs must be addressed when preparing elderly persons for relocation from one residence to another?

This volume examines theories of man-environment relations that provide the basis for research required to answer such questions. Following an overview of the field, general theories are placed in the context of aging, focusing on such processes as environmental cognition, cognitive mapping, complexity, privacy, and territoriality. The relationship between theory and applied research is discussed from different perspectives. Finally, the authors expose gaps in current theory and knowledge, pointing the way for future work.

192 pages   hardcover   1982

Coordinating Community Services for the Elderly
The Triage Experience
Joan Quinn, R.N., M.S., _et al.,_ editors

This book presents an innovative system for delivering comprehensive long-term care services to the elderly based on individual need. It addresses the dilemma of how to provide high-quality yet low-cost care while avoiding unnecessary institutionalization.

The authors describe how to set up such a system, including the organization and reimbursement processes, based on their experience as administrators of Triage, Inc., in Connecticut. Nurses working in the project delineate a holistic approach to client assessment and service coordination and monitoring, with illustrative case examples. Finally, social services researchers evaluate the project and its potential for implementation in other regions of the country.

This is a valuable book for all those involved in delivering health services to the elderly, including administrators, planners and policy makers, researchers, geriatric nurses, and social workers.

144 pages   hardcover   1981

The Day Hospital
Organization and Management
Charlotte M. Hamill, M.A., M.S.S.W., editor

A guide to providing services for chronically ill or physically impaired patients who want to remain in the community. Administrators and health practitioners will find valuable suggestions on program content, program planning, fiscal management, space and equipment needs, and staffing patterns for each type of service in a day hospital.

Included for practical adaptation are appendixes with such tools as admission flow charts, admission interview guide and application, transportation map and guidelines, protocols, and sample patient statistics report. With an extensive bibliography of international sources.

192 pages   hardcover   1981